CHIMBORAZO

Chimborazo

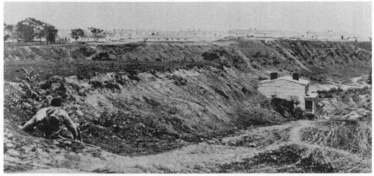

the Confederacy's largest hospital

Carol C. Green

THE UNIVERSITY OF TENNESSEE PRESS

KNOXVILLE

Library of Congress Cataloging-in-Publication Data

Green, Carol Cranmer.
Chimborazo : the Confederacy's largest hospital / Carol C. Green.— 1st ed.
   p. cm.

ISBN 1-57233-316-2

   1. Chimborazo Hospital (Richmond, Va.)
   2. United States—History--Civil War, 1861–1865—Hospitals.
   3. United States—History--Civil War, 1861–1865—Medical care.
   4. Medicine, Military—Confederate States of America—History.
   5. Hospitals—Confederate States of America.
   I. Title.
E625.G74 2004
973.7'76'09755451—dc22   2004012281

Contents

ILLUSTRATIONS

PREFACE

In the years before the Civil War, the most common experiences with serious illness concerned exposure to epidemic diseases such as yellow fever or cholera, or to chronic diseases such as tuberculosis. Americans living in the mid-nineteenth century had a very different view of hospitals than we do today. The term did not bring to mind images of white-clad nurses, antiseptic-smelling hallways, or sterile operating rooms. Instead, they thought of filthy, dimly lit, crowded buildings administered by charities or city governments for those who were destitute, or of the horrors they had read about the military hospitals during the Crimean War of 1853–56, where fatality rates soared to approximately 20 percent in British hospitals and 30 percent in French hospitals.[1] The average American saw hospitals only as places where the chronically ill and poor could go to receive minimal health care if no other options were available to them. Most Americans did not consider the hospital setting healthy or respectable for visits, much less for extended stays.

When the war began, inefficiency and inexperience characterized the treatment of sick and wounded soldiers. One of the quickest realizations, on both sides of the fighting, was the desperate need for the establishment of a systematic plan of medical care, including hospital facilities that could quickly and efficiently treat the growing number of patients who had acquired their maladies while in the patriotic services of their countries. The men were far from home, in situations where the traditional family caregivers were not readily available to care for them. They had acute medical problems that required close medical attention by attendants who knew what to look for and what to do if a life-and-death complication developed. Clearly, a change in the antebellum hospital and its practices was necessary if the army wanted its soldiers to recover sufficiently to return to the fighting and if America's citizens wanted their husbands, fathers, and brothers to return home healthy.

The motivation to change was strong, and the timing was right. "At mid-century," medical historian Charles Rosenberg explained, "every aspect of the relationship between medical knowledge and the hospital was uncertain and subject to future negotiation."[2] America's physicians and hospital reformers were aware of the growing problems with the current hospitals and had begun to work to solve them. The coming of the war placed the efforts of hospital reformers on hold with regard to the public's hospitals but the impetus for change deeply affected the military hospitals that were formed.

Although a great deal of literature examines various features of the Civil War, an important aspect of the war that has received little attention concerns the changes that the Civil War caused in the field of medicine. Most writing on the Civil War only briefly mentions the medical care given to soldiers. If a work refers to the subject at all, it normally features the gore of an amputation done without anesthesia in a haphazard manner by an incompetent surgeon, or some other sensational topic. Although such events did occur, they reveal only one small part of the picture. Before we can claim to understand Civil War medicine, other pieces of the picture must be revealed and fitted into place. One of those other pieces of information concerns life in the military hospitals, on which very little has been written. Surprisingly, even the large dictionaries of Civil War history do not include references to any of the hospitals or medical officers on either side; the sole exceptions are the names of the surgeon generals.

Many works on the history of nineteenth-century medicine essentially ignore the large-scale medical challenge of the Civil War because few great technological advances or new medical theories developed during the war. It is a mistake to focus only on changing technology or new theories as the point at which the practice of medicine changes. Since numerous factors affect the timing of the adoption of new ideas and techniques, rarely is change seen immediately after a "breakthrough." A better approach is to focus on the changing attitudes of the physicians and patients being affected by the technology and existing knowledge.

In addition, many studies have neglected the war because of a hesitancy to link military and civilian medicine, wrongly assuming that what occurred in military settings had no effect on the development of medicine in the private sector. The second reason may be relevant to many wars but cannot apply to the Civil War, which directly affected the lives of most Americans living at the time.

This book, based on an extensive study of the records of Chimborazo Hospital and other primary sources, will attempt to develop a fuller understanding of the Civil War and the history of medicine by carefully examining what occurred at Chimborazo Hospital, the largest and best known hospital in operation during the war. By constructing a picture of life at Chimborazo Hospital this work will describe a major part of a Civil War soldier's life. During the war, of the 600,000 men who fought for the Confederacy "approximately 3,000,000 cases of wounds and disease were cared for by the Medical Corps of the Confederate States Army," according to Richard Boies Stark. "On the average, then," Stark added, "each Confederate soldier was disabled by wounds and sickness about six times during the war."[3] Located just outside of Richmond, Virginia, Chimborazo Hospital treated 77,889 patients from its opening in October 1861 to its surrender to Union troops in April 1865 with a mortality rate of just over 11 percent. Soon after its organization, the hospital became the model on which other Confederate hospitals were based.

Chimborazo Hospital was an innovative facility with well-trained physicians, efficient stewards, caring matrons, and a unique supply system. The hospital's physicians had access to the latest medical knowledge and specialists in Richmond if needed. A review of its records reveals that the medical treatment given to Civil War soldiers in general hospitals was thoughtful and proper. The hospital's clinical reputation grew as it established connections with the Medical College of Virginia and served as the site of several drug and treatment trials requested by the Confederate Medical Department.

This work includes a description of the hospital's facilities, the internal operational dynamics of its management, and the personal side of its staff and patients. Readers will become familiar with life in Chimborazo's wards and how the hospital changed as the war continued. As they meet the people who lived and worked in the hospital, they will celebrate the dedication and gentle wisdom of some figures and frown at the incompetence and apathy of others. The chapters will also reveal some of the major concerns of those at the hospital, including shortages of food and supplies and changes in medical treatment.

After the reader becomes aware of the situation at Chimborazo, it will be clear how this important facility and others like it, in both the North and the South, influenced the development of modern medicine. Civil War hospitals gave doctors experience with treating all classes of patients in an institutional setting. The mission of the war changed the goal of the hospital physician from the management of chronic-care patients to curing acute-care patients quickly—so that they could return to the fighting.

The care that soldiers received in the hospitals improved as the experience of the medical officers and their staffs increased. Doctors gained knowledge from careful observation and trial-and-error techniques and grew increasingly familiar with the existing medical technologies available for diagnosis and treatment. "As the war progressed," noted Alfred Jay Bollet, "we would expect that the accumulated experience and improved organization would result in decreased rates of disease and improved rates of survival from wounds. . . . All these 'expectations' actually did happen."[4] The changes in patient care had implications that lasted far beyond the war.

Although most patients did not understand the new medical ideas or instruments, they did recognize a shift in the attitudes of physicians towards medicine and their patients. The practice of medicine is a highly personalized activity.

When people are sick or injured, the most important aspect of the medical care they receive is how they are treated by the health care workers. In order to be satisfied about the care they receive, patients need to feel that their caregivers are working diligently to solve their health problems. If that need is met, patients will assume that the best technology available was used in their treatment, unless told otherwise. A poor bedside manner can usually only be tolerated in a life-or-death situation with a positive outcome. Even then, the patient and his family do not soon forget how they were treated by the medical staff. They might respect the skill of the staff, but that will never allow them to excuse a bad personal situation without complaint. The extensive support staffs that developed in hospitals, including the presence of female matrons and nurses, helped to reinforce the positive image of hospitals and contributed to the pleasantness of the hospital experience by improving aspects of patient care beyond the medical realm.

During the war thousands of patients were exposed to hospitals in which they were treated with respect and provided with good medical care in a comfortable and safe environment. Although its institutional lifespan was relatively short, Chimborazo Hospital affected the development of modern medicine by directly exposing a large number of soldiers to successful medical treatment in a large institutional setting. The success of hospitals such as Chimborazo began to change Americans' perceptions of hospitals and prompted people to see value in large medical institutions. The war's large medical facilities provided interesting models that effectively dealt with the war's medical and bureaucratic challenges and had many similarities to the modern paying hospitals of the twentieth century.

ACKNOWLEDGMENTS

This book is the product of many years of work and effort. I would like to express my appreciation to the many individuals who helped me develop my understanding about Chimborazo. Dr. Ronald Rainger, my graduate mentor, provided valuable insight and attention to detail during the dissertation stage of this work. The staff of the University of Tennessee Press did a remarkable job with the editing process. The archivists at the National Archives, the Richmond National Battlefield Park, the Museum of the Confederacy, and the Thompkins-McCaw Library in Richmond were also very helpful with helping me locate information and photographs.

My husband, Robert, receives my deepest gratitude for his help along every step of the process. His constant love and encouragement motivated me to do my best; his patience enabled me to immerse myself in my work; his curious and insightful questions helped me to understand many facets of Chimborazo that I would have otherwise missed.

CHAPTER 1

The Organization of the Confederate Medical Department and Chimborazo Hospital

When the Civil War began, Americans in both the North and the South hoped that the conflict would end quickly and result in few deaths. The medical departments of the Union and Confederate armies were small, poorly funded, and had very little authority. As we know now, the conflict lasted four long years and was responsible for the deaths of almost 620,000 Americans (360,000 Union and 260,000 Confederate). As the fighting continued and intensified, both the Union and Confederate armies realized the importance of a good medical corps: soldiers had to be healthy to march and fight.

The Union army had a small medical department in place when the war started, but it needed to be radically expanded and strengthened to meet the challenges of the war. Elderly and cautious surgeons general and extremely low budgets limited the department's effectiveness in 1861. "The first two surgeons general could think only in terms of a peacetime army of twelve thousand to sixteen thousand men," explained medical historian John Duffy. "Colonel Thomas Lawson, a veteran of the War of 1812 already in his eighties, considered medical books an extravagance."[1] Lawson's replacement, Clement A. Finley, "had spent a lifetime in the army making do with as little as possible. . . . Conditioned to the army's emphasis on seniority and the rituals of peacetime life, he simply could not cope with an emergency situation."[2] The following year, Secretary of War Edwin M. Stanton appointed William Alexander Hammond as the new surgeon general. Hammond quickly began to reform his department, radically expanding

1

the budget, forming an ambulance corps, and basing appointments and promotions on merit rather than seniority. The United States Sanitary Commission (USSC), established on July 9, 1861, also played a major role in the reforms and success of the Union army's medical department. The USSC sought to help the medical department to preserve and maintain the health of the troops by conducting medical inspections of camps, providing emergency supplies, and recruiting nurses, cooks, and other peripheral personnel to serve in Union hospitals.[3]

The Confederacy had no existing medical department, so it based its system closely on the Union model, with a few exceptions. Because it had no medical corps already in place, the senior officers could be selected on the basis of merit rather than seniority without causing a great deal of controversy. "Whereas the Union army relied largely upon state-appointed regimental surgeons," wrote Duffy, "the Confederate government directly commissioned its approximately 5,800 medical officers."[4] Physicians who had considerable knowledge and experience were designated as surgeons. Less seasoned doctors became assistant surgeons. The surgeons assigned to positions of authority, such as hospital administration, were placed there deliberately because of their medical reputations and personal strengths, rather than their rank, length of service, or political connections. A review of the leadership in the Confederate Medical Department and the major Confederate hospitals in Richmond reveals very little turnover. The Confederacy had only one surgeon general over the course of the war—compared to four in the Union medical department. The medical director positions in the South also saw scant change. Little motivation existed for a physician in the Confederate army to change assignments. Because physicians intended to remain in the army only for the duration of the war, transfers for purposes of furthering a military career did not apply. Confederate medical regulations did not allow for promotions until an assistant surgeon had served for five years. By the time any ambitious assistant surgeons could consider this as an option, the Confederacy's victory was in doubt.

The continuity of the Confederate Medical Department differed from the Union system, which operated with career medical officers seeking promotions and high-profile civilian organizations such as the United States Sanitary Commission (USSC) criticizing some physicians and lobbying for others to gain important assignments. Four surgeons general served during the war years, and many hospital administrators rarely stayed for more than one or two years.[5] Of course, family connections and politics could have affected the appointment and assignments of the Confederacy's surgeons, but the lack of a group such as the USSC allowed those physicians to focus on the job at hand instead of the politics. The resulting continuity of leadership greatly aided the Confederate Medical Department in making its part of the war effort as effective as possible.

Other features of a newly created Medical Department also contributed to the Confederacy's success. Because of the lack of an established bureaucracy, Confederate medical officers had less red tape to deal with, in contrast to their counterparts in the Union medical department. Also, the lack of a distinction between the regular army and the volunteer corps contributed to the sense of single-minded purpose within the Medical Department. The confidence and flexibility that resulted from the newness of the Confederate Medical Department encouraged the formation of large hospitals such as Chimborazo and gave its administrators the means to operate them successfully.

The Confederate army's Medical Department was created on February 26, 1861, when the Confederate Congress passed the Act for the Establishment and Organization of a General Staff for the Army of the Confederate States of America. As H. H. Cunningham explained, "This measure, passed eight days after the inauguration of Jefferson Davis, provided for a medical department of one surgeon general, four surgeons, and six assistant surgeons."[6] At this initial point, the concept of the Confederate Medical Department was to help coordinate the activities of the medical staffs provided by the states. Each Southern state appointed a surgeon general for its military. Dr. David C. DeLeon, said to be "a member of one of Mobile, Alabama's most distinguished families," was appointed as the surgeon general for his home state in February 1861 and given the rank of colonel.[7] Because Montgomery served as the Confederacy's capital in the early months of the war, DeLeon was looked to as a central figure in the initial organization of the Confederate Medical Department.

The position of surgeon general of the Confederacy remained open until March 16, 1861, when Jefferson Davis and others convinced Dr. Samuel Preston Moore to accept the position, a move that placed Moore directly under the supervision of the secretary of war and gave him the rank and privileges of a brigadier general of the cavalry.[8] Described as "a handsome man, tall and erect, of impressive military bearing," Samuel Preston Moore was one of three United States Army surgeons who had resigned their commissions when the Civil War broke out.[9] His many years of medical experience in a military setting made him an obvious choice to lead the Confederate Medical Department.

Born and raised in Charleston, South Carolina, Moore graduated from the Medical College of South Carolina on March 8, 1834. In 1835 he became an assistant surgeon in the United States Army. Over the next decade he served at various western posts—including Fort Leavenworth, Kansas; Fort Des Moines, Iowa; and Fort Gibson, Missouri—as well as at several forts in Florida. During the Mexican War (1846–48), Moore was stationed at Camargo, south of the Rio Grande River, where he served with Jefferson Davis. In April 1849 Moore was promoted to surgeon with the rank of major while serving at Jefferson Barracks, Missouri. In 1855, after serving at posts in Oregon, Texas, and New York, he was assigned to the United States Military Academy at West Point, where he remained until April 1860. He then served as the medical purveyor in New Orleans until the Civil War

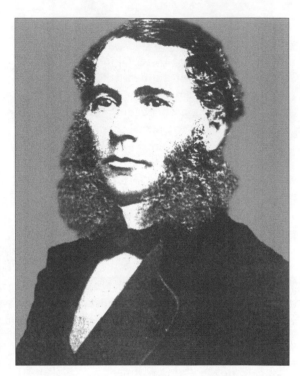

Samuel Preston Moore
(1813–1889), c. 1845. From Ira
Rutkow, "Samuel Preston
Moore," in Regulations for the
Army of the Confederate States,
By Order of the Surgeon General
(1862; reprint, San Francisco:
Norman Publishing, 1992), i.

broke out. After resigning his commission in the U.S. Army, he moved to Little Rock, Arkansas, to open a general medical practice, and he remained there until beginning his work as surgeon general in July.[10]

Moore's duties did not fully begin until after the Fort Sumter incident prompted Virginia and the other states in the upper South to secede. At that point, the separate military forces of the states were absorbed by the Confederacy, and Virginia invited the Confederate government to move its capital from Montgomery to Richmond. On May 21 the Confederate Congress accepted the invitation and planned to meet in Richmond on July 20.[11] On July 30, 1861, Moore was ordered to Richmond to begin his duties as acting surgeon general, which included, according to H. H. Cunningham, "the administrative details of the medical department, the government of hospitals, the regulation of the duties of surgeons and assistant surgeons, and the appointment of acting medical officers, when needed, for local or detached service."[12]

One by one, Moore addressed the many problems that he encountered with orderliness and dedication, determined to mold his department into a highly disciplined organization similar to that of the U.S. Army he had left only a few months before. His thoroughness, attention to detail, and stern sense of discipline contributed to his success as an organizer and administrator, although those characteristics did not make him a popular official. Surgeon Pyre Porcher, a close associate of Moore, revealed his opinion of the surgeon general in an article after the war:

> A native of Charleston and a man trained in the army, with all its formality, he may have contracted certain habitudes which deprived his manners . . . of that softness and suavity which are used in the representative democracies and in all non military communities.
>
> Within his domain, which was an extensive one, he had absolute power and the fiat of an autocrat; the Emperor of the Russians was not more autocratic. He commanded and it was done. He stood *in terrorem* over the surgeon, whatever his rank, or wherever he might be—from Richmond to the trans-Mississippi. Although appearing to be cold and forbidding, we do not feel that Surgeon Moore was cruel, arbitrary, or insensitive to conviction.[13]

Another officer stated, "He was a man of great brusqueness of manner and gave offense to many who called on him, whatever their business, and without any regard to their station or rank, though he was an able executive officer, and I believe an efficient and impartial one."[14] It must be remembered that most of the medical officers Moore dealt with had little if any previous training in military discipline or procedure, and it seems evident that the surgeon general was more concerned with efficiency than polite conversation. J. Boulware, a South Carolinian who served as a hospital steward and later as a contract surgeon, appears to have summed up Moore's personae when he wrote, "I found the Surgeon General quite a pleasant talking gentleman, yet he spoke to the point freely."[15]

The largest single problem Moore faced when he became surgeon general was adequately caring for the increasing number of sick and wounded men in the Confederate army. Moore's administrative talent quickly revealed itself as he began to expand and organize his department in order to care for those soldiers. The large number of casualties at the Battle of Manassas, which occurred on July 21, 1861, just before Moore arrived in Richmond, dramatically illustrated the scope of this problem: 1,582 Confederate soldiers were killed and 387 were wounded. This number of casualties was by far the greatest that Americans had seen in one battle. As battles were fought, the wounded soldiers were transported to Richmond as soon as possible so that the troops' movements would not be slowed by the men in the army's field hospitals. Richmond became the medical center of the Confederacy for many reasons. Most important, wrote Clifford Dowdey, "as Richmond was in proximity to all the fighting in the east, more than 60 per cent of the Confederate wounded passed through its hospitals."[16] Also, Richmond was the largest city in the region, the Confederate capital, and a transportation hub with road, railroad, and ship access.

Besides the large numbers of wounded, thousands of sick soldiers also needed hospital beds. "On August 17, 1861," noted Cunningham, "General Joseph E. Johnston, at Manassas, reported 4,809 sick of 18,178 present."[17] Most soldiers, because of ignorance or laziness or both, neglected personal and camp cleanliness and prepared their foods carelessly. Dysentery and typhoid fever quickly resulted from the improper placement and neglect of latrines. Also, the vast majority of Southerners lived in a rural environment and had been exposed to only a limited number of infantile diseases, such as measles and chickenpox. As the men of the South came to northern Virginia and joined their local regiments to the Confederacy's main armies, their lack of immunity resulted in epidemic outbreaks of these sicknesses. As Cunningham reported, "Paul Fitzsimons Eve . . . who served as surgeon general of Tennessee and in the Gate City Hospital of Atlanta during the Civil War, concluded that 'at the organization of the army, one town regiment was more efficient than two or even three from the country.'"[18]

Richmond was not ready for the large numbers of sick and wounded who were being transported in daily from the army's camps and front lines. The city had been filled even before the fighting had begun. The local diarist Mary Boykin Chesnut noted on June, 12, 1861: "Richmond is crowded & the hotels are overflowing."[19] In 1860 Richmond had only five small facilities that provided medical care. Bellevue Hospital, Richmond's first private hospital, which had opened in June 1854, had a normal bed capacity of fifty-one patients; the Medical College of Virginia's infirmary could care for seventy-five patients; and the St. Francis Infirmary, located on the northwest edge of the city, had room for thirty patients. The other two facilities were Richmond's Almshouse and the Main Street Hospital, a small facility that provided care for free blacks and slaves.[20]

In June 1861 the Confederate Medical Department began to expand hospital capacity for the soldiers by renting Richmond's newly built Almshouse, designating it as General Hospital No. 1 for the duration of the war. This large brick building, said to have been "the only building in Richmond adapted to hospital purposes," was capable of holding five hundred patients. Dr. Charles Bell Gibson, who had served briefly as Virginia's surgeon general before the consolidation of the medical departments, was named the surgeon-in-charge of the facility. A Confederate surgeon would later state, "At that time this hospital was the best in the Confederacy. Besides an excellent corps of surgeons, there were the gentle Catholic 'Sisters.'"[21]

The limited hospital space prompted the army's sick and wounded to be placed in any available building—hotels, factories, warehouses, stores, taverns, churches, and private homes all served as makeshift hospitals. "Samuel P. Day, an English observer, found about fifteen hundred patients being cared for in twelve Richmond hospitals after the first clash at Manassas, and many were being treated elsewhere," Cunningham wrote. "According to Day, only 'a fractional part of the sick and wounded' were in the hospitals."[22] Having to use hotels, warehouses, and other existing buildings for hospital purposes alarmed Surgeon General Moore and other physicians who were aware of the horrors that British soldiers had suffered in similar buildings during the Crimean War. The lack of ventilation and cleanliness encouraged the spread of contagious diseases, the distribution of medical personnel and supplies would be practically impossible, and the use of these buildings as hospitals would most likely render them unfit for further use.

It quickly became evident that the Medical Department and its facilities had to be radically expanded to meet the needs of the Confederate troops. According to Cunningham, "Moore . . . advised the Secretary of the Treasury, who was in charge of arrangements for establishing the public offices in Richmond, that it was 'impossible to transact the business of this bureau (connected most intimately with the welfare of the Army in the field) in one single room, crowded to overflowing with employees, soldiers, and visitors on business.'"[23] The request for more space was granted; the surgeon general's offices were moved and placed in the same building as the offices of the war department.

Moore's concern about the limited available hospital space deepened in October, when General Johnston informed Moore that the large number of sick and wounded in his regiment field hospitals was making it difficult to move his troops quickly or easily. He requested that room be made in Richmond so the patients could be transported there. Since the hospitals in the city were already overflowing, Moore was unsure of what he could do. He discovered an answer during a conversation with Dr. James Brown McCaw, a respected Richmond physician and professor at the Medical College of Virginia. McCaw later reported their discussion in an 1897 interview.

> Surgeon-General S. P. Moore . . . came to see me, and asked what could be done? I was not in the service at the time, but had enlisted in a cavalry company, which was being organized and equipped at our own expense, so I determined to do what I could to meet the emergency. . . . I made the suggestion that we should take the hill forming the eastern prolong of Broad street, and use it for hospital purposes.[24]

Until this decision, the hill had been used to organize the troops coming into Richmond. "All trains brought troops from some part of Virginia or from other Southern states, who were marched to the camps—one at the Fair Grounds . . . , one at Howard's Grove . . . , one on Chimborazo Hill."[25]

On October 9, 1861, Moore ordered McCaw to organize and direct such a hospital, which, at the suggestion of McCaw, would be named Chimborazo Hospital, after the popular name for the Virginia plateau on which it would stand. The name "Chimborazo" refers to a 20,702-foot volcano in central Ecuador that is part of the Andes mountain chain. Richmond legend maintains that some international traveler christened the hill east of the city Chimborazo because of its likeness to the South American volcano, easily seen from out at sea. A brewery had dug cellars in the Richmond hill to store beer. At the top of the cellars was a hole that acted as a chimney. As a Richmond newspaper reported, any fire in the cellar would cause "billows of smoke [to come] through making the hill look like a miniature Vesuvius."[26]

The site selected by McCaw was ideal for hospital purposes. Located east of Richmond, "Chimborazo Hill" was an elevated plateau of nearly forty acres that "swept to a high bluff overlooking the [James] river. It was sunny in the winter and the coolest spot in Richmond in the summer. Residential streets on Church Hill did not extend eastward beyond the wide ravine of Bloody Run Gully . . . and the hospital, built east of the ravine, enjoyed the physical atmosphere of the country."[27] The York River Railroad passed along the base of the hill, allowing easy access when necessary. From the heights of the plateau, the hospital's view was impressive. Richmond lay toward the west; toward the east were forests and cultivated fields, and to the south one could see the busy James River. Before McCaw chose the Chimborazo plateau as the site for his hospital, only two buildings were located on the hill: a large house owned by Richard Laughton and a small office building.[28]

Chimborazo Hospital developed into the best-known hospital in the Confederacy and the largest hospital anywhere in the world at that time. At McCaw's request, Moore designated the "Hospital on the Hill," as it was quickly nicknamed, to be an independent army post with McCaw as its commandant or "surgeon-in-chief." It was organized into five divisions, each a separate hospital led by a "surgeon-in-charge."

McCaw quickly began work on the monumental task of organizing Chimborazo Hospital. McCaw leased the Laughton house, located immediately north of where the hospital wards were to be built. It served as the hospital's main headquarters, holding the offices of the surgeon-in-chief, the surgeons-in-charge, and the other necessary offices of the post. The earliest surviving document relating to the institution is a letter from the medical purveyor addressed to McCaw, dated October 15, 1861. This note told McCaw that his invoice for hospital supplies had been turned over to the Quartermaster's Office for transportation on October 13. It gave McCaw instructions to report back to the Purveyor's Office when the supplies arrived at Chimborazo with information about what had been received and whether the received supplies corresponded with the invoice sent.[29] Other records from October included a special requisition sent to the quartermaster from McCaw, asking for ten barrels of lime, and an order directing T. Braxton, an assistant surgeon, to "report to the Acting Surgeon Gen. for duty in the Hospital in this City under charge of Dr. McKaw [sic]."[30]

Construction quickly began on the wards for the patients as well as the other buildings needed for a large hospital. McCaw remembered the construction period as follows:

> We bought out the Grants, Mayos and other large tobacco manufacturers whose vocation was practically at an end for the period of the war, and made use of the boilers from their factories for making soup in our soup-houses, and the large supply of splendidly seasoned wood for making tobacco boxes . . . supplied us with materials for making beds and other furniture. We took charge of the hands employed in these tobacco factories and used them in doing the manual labor incident to building, etc., in our hospital construction.[31]

Undressed two-inch-thick pine planks, whitewashed with lime, were used to build the one-story wards, which were eighty feet long by twenty-eight feet wide with sides seven feet tall. The walls' boards were nailed on vertically, and the crevices were then covered with wooden strips. Shingled roofs topped the buildings. On the side of each ward were three doors, two-and-a-half feet wide by six feet tall on each side, and ten windows, about two feet square, which could be closed with sliding wooden shutters. Each ward was finished with a rough plank floor, then divided into two apartments by a low partition set lengthwise.[32] Four rows of wooden bunks and one or two centrally located stoves furnished the

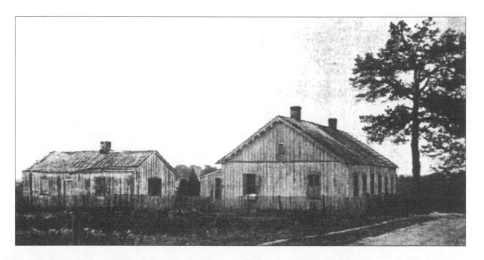

An example of a ward at Winder Hospital. This building, similar in construction to Chimborazo's wards, was used as a residence in the 1890s. From Robert Waitt, *Confederate Military Hospitals in Richmond* (Richmond, Va.: City of Richmond, 1964), 33.

wards. These wards were built to hold thirty-two patients each. By mid-1862, ninety-eight patient wards had been constructed.

These buildings were not meant to be permanent structures. From the description, it is most likely that balloon construction was used to build Chimborazo's wards. First used in the United States in the 1830s, this type of frame substituted thin plates and studs for more sturdy and costly mortising and joining. As Nathan Rosenberg noted, "[I]ts lightness and simplicity—the house was essentially nailed together with light 2-inch x 4-inch studs—sharply reduced the total labor requirements of construction and made it possible to substitute relatively unskilled labor for the skilled carpenter. What [the design] lacked in elegance was more than compensated for by its highly utilitarian qualities and, above all, by its cheapness."[33] The balloon method of construction was still relatively uncommon in the 1860s; it only became firmly established when it was used widely for quick reconstruction after the Great Chicago Fire of 1871. However, it was perfect for the wards at Chimborazo. The slaves who were used to build the wards had previously worked in Richmond's tobacco warehouses and thus had little or no construction experience. This type of construction required little training, could be put together in a very short time, and was inexpensive.

The wards were erected in rows and were positioned so that the wind, which normally blew from the northwest to the southeast, would blow through the windows and doors for maximum ventilation. Such attention to detail is admirable for a facility that was constructed so quickly. "[L]aticed [*sic*] structures over the combs of the roofs" also helped keep fresh air in the wards.[34] The placement of the wards in the pavilion design also aided ventilation. Experience from the Crimean War in the 1850s taught that adequate ventilation was critical to good hospital facilities. Physicians commonly believed that disease was spread by unhealthy or contaminated air, called "effluvia" or "miasmas," which floated through the air, potentially infecting those who breathed it with fevers or disease.

Avenues forty feet wide separated the rows; narrower alleys ten to twelve feet wide ran between the wards in the rows. Several of the outside wards were built with a deviation from the rectangular arrangement because of their proximity to the edge of the hill, which dropped off sharply into Bloody Run.

The design and placement of its wards made Chimborazo the first pavilion hospital to operate in the United States. Historical records do not reveal whether the idea to build Chimborazo Hospital on the pavilion plan came from Dr. McCaw, but we do know that he was the individual who suggested the location of the hospital, which was perfect for the pavilion design. Such a large undertaking certainly had to have the approval of Moore. Actually, it matters little who thought of using the pavilion plan; the important thing was that its implementation at Chimborazo Hospital set it apart, even from the beginning, as an innovative facility.

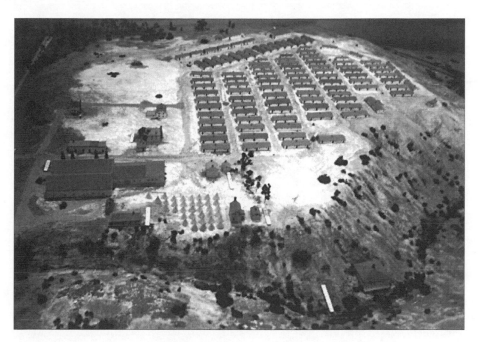

A model of Chimborazo Hospital showing building placement. Photograph by Robert Green. The model is on display at Richmond National Battlefield Park Headquarters, Richmond, Virginia.

The pavilion design had first received attention in France at the end of the eighteenth century when the construction of the new Hotel Dieu was being discussed. The plan called for a number of one-story wards, designed and placed to facilitate maximum ventilation. However, the pavilion plan received little widespread attention until the 1850s, when Florence Nightingale returned from her experiences in the Crimean War and began her crusade to change many features of hospitals. Her opinions, printed in *Notes on Hospitals,* along with a series of reports released by the British Parliament, including that of the Commission on the Sanitary Condition of Barracks and Hospitals in 1861, supported the idea of hospitals "composed of separate, isolated pavilions with large airy wards, well lit and ventilated by windows along both long sides."[35] The most prominent example of the implementation of the pavilion design in England was Herbert Hospital at Woolwich, near London; its construction began in 1859 but was not completed until 1864. The following year, the first permanent American hospital to use the design, the Hospital of the Protestant Episcopal Church in Philadelphia, began its construction, which continued until 1874.[36]

The pavilion design quickly became the style of hospital architecture preferred by American physicians. Surgeon Charles S. Tripler, the medical director of the Union's Army of the Potomac, explained why he and so many of his contemporaries favored the design: "They admit of more perfect ventilation, can be kept in better police, are more convenient for the sick and wounded and their attendants, admit of a ready distribution of patients into the proper classes, and are cheaper."[37]

The patient wards were supplied from a central storehouse, conveniently located in the middle of the rectangular design of the pavilions. The other buildings of the hospital were located north and east of the patient wards. The larger buildings included the headquarters office, the kitchens, the huge bakery, the soaphouse, the five icehouses, and a large stable. Numerous smaller buildings housed the hospital's staff, the chapel, and the shops of the carpenters, blacksmiths, and apothecaries. The guardhouse and the hospital's five deadhouses sat on the northern perimeter of the hospital's grounds. A brewery used by the hospital was located just outside the hospital's grounds. A large dairy and a sawmill used by the hospital were located on Williamsburg Avenue, just across the York River Railroad. The hospital also included a large vegetable garden two and a half miles away and Franklin Stearn's "Tree Hill" farm, on which the hospital's many goats and milk cows were kept. At the end of the war over 150 structures made up the Chimborazo complex.[38]

The hospital's water supply was safely located on the top of the hill. "Morley and Cornelius, slave welldiggers employed by Chimborazo, apparently helped dig five deep wells which were watered by three good springs."[39] The wells conveniently lay near the ends of the wide streets. The hospital also had two other wells and two springs. In late January 1862 the Quartermaster's Department authorized the construction of a bathhouse at Chimborazo, which was soon built on the western side of grounds, slightly down the hill. The latrines were farther down the hill and apparently drained into Bloody Run.

All of the activity at Chimborazo did not go unnoticed. The *Richmond Whig* discussed the events in its November 1 edition:

> The plateau overlooking Rocketts, known as Chimborazo Hill, has
> recently been covered with one story wooden buildings, presenting
> the appearance of a large Danish village. These buildings were erected
> by direction of the Quartermaster General of the C.S.A. . . . we believe,
> to use them for hospital purposes. Two or three hundred sick soldiers
> are already quartered at the place.[40]

Chimborazo Hospital admitted its first patients in October 1861. After that, the hospital grew quickly. On December 5 Moore instructed McCaw "to make pro-

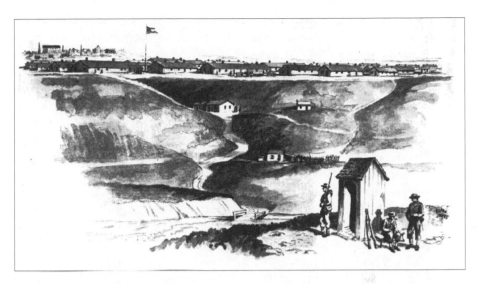

Drawing of Chimborazo Hospital as sketched by an observer in 1862. From Robert Waitt, *Confederate Military Hospitals in Richmond* (Richmond, Va.: City of Richmond, 1964).

vision for 1000 convalescents, in addition to the number of sick in [the] hospital." In the same letter Moore revealed that the number of sick men currently at Chimborazo was 1,200.[41]

A variety of patients filled Chimborazo during the first year of its operation. The initial idea was to use Chimborazo primarily for convalescent patients and as an overflow area to relieve the burdens of the hospitals in Richmond. On March 18 Moore wrote McCaw, authorizing him to transfer patients to their appropriate state hospitals when the patients had notes from those facilities stating that there was room for them.[42] There are many examples of letters in 1862 from hospital administrators of the various state hospitals in Richmond to McCaw, advising him that they had room for patients from their states. A typical example of this correspondence is a letter from the secretary of the Louisiana Hospital to McCaw: "[W]e have 10 vacant beds which we would like to fill with sick & not convalescent patients, provided they are in your opinion able to be transferred with proficity— we have some 75 or 80 patients from other States besides Louisiana which, as they are mostly convalescent, we would be more than happy to exchange with you."[43]

The conditions in Richmond continued to be crowded in 1862, even though Chimborazo housed over 3,000 patients—more than half of the sick in Richmond. On April 2 Moore told McCaw that Chimborazo "must receive as many sick as the hospital can accommodate. The number must go up to 3500 or 3700, which the hospital has accommodated. The men must be crowded for a few days." McCaw responded by forwarding the order to his surgeons-in-charge, telling them that each hospital would have to take 40 men: "[T]he men sent tonight must be taken and put on the floor if other accommodations cannot be given. They will leave them here, and say we must take them."[44] However, McCaw evidently put his foot down when ordered to take more patients. On April 21 Moore ordered the hospitals in town to "take all patients sent to [you] by Mr. Peters, the Master of Ambulances. The crowded state cannot be avoided. This must occur until the buildings being fitted are completed." This order did not apply to Chimborazo Hospital. Instead, the surgeons-in-charge were instructed to notify Peters every morning about the number of patients that could be accommodated.[45]

As crowded conditions continued to threaten the effective medical treatment of Confederate troops, Moore established more hospitals. By the summer of 1862, Moore had organized several other facilities including General Hospital No. 5 (formerly a dry goods store) with 100 patients and General Hospital No. 8 (formerly the Saint Charles Hotel) with 460 patients.[46] However, the sick and wounded continued to pour into Richmond faster than the Medical Department could act, and the demand for hospital space still far exceeded the amount available. Moore knew that as the weather became warmer and the rainy season ended, the fighting would intensify, resulting in more wounded to care for. In 1862 he began to establish hospitals in towns away from Richmond to which convalescent patients could be transferred when needed. This relieved some of the pressure on the city. Since the patients would be transferred by railcar, these hospitals were located in the larger towns along the railroad, such as Danville, Gordonville, and Lynchburg. Not surprisingly, in April 1862 Moore ordered McCaw to help him with the task. Chimborazo's founder was to "proceed with as little delay as practicable to Danville for the purpose of establishing hospitals in that city." McCaw was to select enough factories to accommodate 5,000 patients and "make the proper requisitions on the Qr. Master of the post for the proper hiring, cleaning, and fitting of these buildings." After carrying out these orders, McCaw was to resume his duties at Chimborazo.[47]

Another way to expand hospital space was to construct and organize other hospital complexes based on the innovative pattern Chimborazo had established. On April 10, 1862, Chimborazo's sister hospital, Winder Hospital, admitted its first patients. Located on twenty-five acres on the western edge of Richmond on Cary street, Camp Winder, as it was often called, constituted wards set in the pavilion design and organized into five divisions plus a tent division, very similar to Chimborazo. Twenty-seven-year-old Alexander Lane, a native of Louisiana, served as the surgeon-in-chief of Winder throughout the war. From 1862 to 1865 Camp Winder treated 76,123 soldiers, and at times its census temporarily rose above Chimborazo's.[48]

Although Moore's efforts to open new hospitals helped the situation, the battles around Richmond in the summer of 1862 renewed the problem of where to house and care for the Confederacy's wounded. The Battle of Seven Pines, which was fought near the Chickahominy River less than six miles from Richmond, occurred on May 31 and June 1 and resulted in heavy casualties: 6,184 Confederate soldiers were listed as dead, wounded, or missing.[49] The Seven Days Battles, which included five major encounters between Union and Confederate troops from June 26 to July 1, resulted in 20,614 Confederate casualties. These battles were fought east of Richmond, making Chimborazo Hospital the closest medical facility.[50]

The only other large hospital on that side of Richmond was Howard's Grove Hospital, located northeast of Richmond along Mechanicsville Turnpike. A popular Richmond picnic site before the war, Howard's Grove received its first patients on June 26, the day of the Mechanicsville battle. Its buildings were constructed according to the pavilion model employed at Chimborazo and Winder, but its single division allowed the facility to hold considerably fewer patients than its sister hospitals.[51]

Even with the large capacities of the pavilion hospitals, Richmond continued to be crowded. John B. Jones, a war clerk in the Confederate War Department in Richmond, stated, "There are fifty hospitals in the city, fast filling with the sick and wounded. I have seen men in my office and walking in the streets whose arms have been amputated within the last three days. The realization of a great victory seems to give them strength."[52] Another resident of Richmond, Mrs. Sally Putnam, wrote the following to describe the situation after the Seven Days' Battles:

> The month of July of 1862 can never be forgotten in Richmond. We lived in one immense hospital, and breathed the vapors of the charnel house. . . . Every family received the bodies of the wounded or dead of their friends, and every house was a house of mourning or a private hospital. . . . Sickening odors filled the atmosphere, and soldiers' funerals were passing at every moment. . . . Our best and brightest young men were passing away.[53]

Although the summer of 1862 probably saw the most patients directly admitted from the field to Richmond hospitals, the capital continued to serve as the medical hub for the battles fought in the Virginia area. As soon as patients could be transported away from the field hospitals and smaller general hospitals, they were usually sent to Richmond for care before being transferred to a convalescent hospital to recuperate.

Throughout the rest of 1862, whenever it seemed that the city began to catch its breath and empty its hospital wards, another major battle would fill them again. The Second Battle of Manassas in late August was followed by Lee's advance into Maryland and the Battle at Antietam in September. Several thousand more casualties arrived in Richmond via train in mid-December after the Battle of Fredericksburg. The large number of patients, in addition to the expanded regular population and the increasing numbers of refugees to the city, made the winter of 1862–63 a hard one. The crowding in the city and the scarcity of supplies strengthened Moore's resolve to move as many patients as possible to areas outside the city.

In early 1863 Moore began a reorganization process. He began closing the smaller private hospitals and makeshift general hospitals; only a very few small hospitals were allowed to remain open. Generally, hospitals with fewer than a hundred beds were closed first. Interestingly, Moore closed these hospitals with an element of decorum. In a February letter written to Medical Director William Carrington, Moore acknowledged, "[T]he better plan [than that of removing patients and property from the private hospitals] appears to be to let these private hospitals alone for the present. As the ladies are very desirous of attending to sick soldiers, they should be gratified." Moore further instructed Carrington to find out how many beds were available in these facilities, so as to "keep them filled up" until they were to be closed.[54] By March of 1864, thirty-five hospitals in Richmond had closed.

One exception to the closures was Robertson Hospital, operated by Sally L. Tompkins, a Richmond citizen. Tompkins paid all the expenses to keep her twenty-two-bed hospital running from June 1862 to February 1865. For her efforts she received a captain's commission from the Confederacy, making her the only female officer in the Confederate army appointed in the Civil War. Since Tompkins's hospital required no funding, passed the inspections of the Confederate Medical Department, and had a better success rate than most other Confederate hospitals, Moore saw no reason to close the institution.[55]

The small hospitals that had been closed were replaced with new and expanded facilities in the large camp hospitals. Jackson Hospital, located west of Hollywood Cemetery not far from Camp Winder, opened on June 29, 1863, and consisted of four divisions.[56] The capacity of Howard's Grove tripled with the addition of two new divisions. Beginning in late 1862, Moore designated Howard's Grove as the smallpox hospital for the Richmond area; it treated some civilians as well as military personnel. Wards A, B, C, E, and F housed mainly smallpox patients; Ward D contained some smallpox patients but mostly rubeola patients. The few patients who were being treated for other sicknesses or wounds were usually transferred to other hospitals; many were sent to General Hospital No. 1 in Lynchburg.[57]

Throughout 1861 and 1862, patients had been sent to Chimborazo as an overflow area. When McCaw became aware of available space in the state hospitals in Richmond, he could transfer patients to those facilities, but as the smaller hospitals closed, the role of the large pavilion hospitals changed.[58] In July 1863 all military hospitals in the Richmond area were reapportioned: hospitals were specifically designated to treat patients of only one state. As Carrington informed McCaw:

The sick & wounded will be sent to the Hospitals as dicated [*sic*] for their respective States when not injurious to themselves or greatly inconvenient to the service, in which case they will be sent to those indicated as Confederate Hospitals on account of their proximity to the Receiving & Distributing Hospital. Only in case of the receipt of large number of wounded (within a short period) will this arrangement be departed from.[59]

Patients began to be routinely distributed among different hospitals according to which state they called home.

TABLE 1
Proper Disbursement of Patients among Confederate Hospitals in Richmond after 1863

State	Hospital
Alabama	General Hospitals No. 20 & 21
Arkansas	General Hospital No. 25
Florida	General Hospital No. 11
Georgia	Chimborazo No. 2, Jackson, Winder
Kentucky	Chimborazo, Winder
Louisiana	Jackson
Maryland	Chimborazo No. 2
Mississippi	Winder
Missouri	Chimborazo
North Carolina	Jackson, General Hospitals No. 22 & 24
South Carolina	Jackson, Winder
Tennessee	Chimborazo, Winder
Texas	General Hospital No. 25
Virginia	Chimborazo No. 1
Officers	General Hospitals No. 4 & 10
Patients with Smallpox, Measles, etc.	Howard's Grove Hospital
Patients with Mental Illness	General Hospital No. 13
Prisoners Needing Medical Attention	General Hospital No. 13

Once the distribution of patients by state had begun, the Confederate hospital system around Richmond finally seemed stabilized. By that point, Richmond had five large hospital complexes. The network of hospitals in towns not far from Richmond by rail could relieve much of the pressure when the battles occurred closer to Richmond and increased the need for empty patient beds. The major leadership in the Medical Department and in the hospitals had been chosen and most would remain set for the duration of the war. The physicians of the Confederate Medical Department finally had time to devote to the day-to-day treatment of the patients under their care and administration of the facilities under their charge. This time of optimism would not last long, however. By 1863 the war effort began to take its toll on the resources of the Confederacy. The shortages of various items and other practical concerns suffered by the South as it slowly lost its strength to the more wealthy and populous North renewed the challenge for those in the Confederate Medical Department and limited their abilities to improve medical care as much as they would have liked.

In many ways, the challenges faced by the Confederate Medical Department testify to its success. From the medical records that exist, it is remarkable that little difference existed between the mortality statistics and medical practices of the Union and Confederate medical departments—especially when one factors in the huge contributions of supplies, manpower, and other support that the United States Sanitary Commission and similar agencies provided to the Union. The advantages that the Confederacy had through its consistent leadership and pragmatic, flexible approach to the organization and management of medical facilities perhaps aided the Confederate effort more than is readily apparent.

The formation of Chimborazo Hospital and its success illustrates the remarkable character of the Confederate Medical Department. Employing a new and controversial hospital architecture would have been much more difficult for the Union medical department of 1861. The North's first two surgeons general did not see the need for wide-scale hospital construction and would not have approved the innovative design. It was not until William Hammond adopted the construction of pavilion hospitals as a pet project in 1862 that the Union medical department began to address the large-scale problem of providing enough hospital facilities. Even then, with Hammond's diligent personal attention, the first pavilion-style Union hospitals did not open until the end of 1862.[60] The idea of such a large medical complex as Chimborazo was, in itself, a radical departure from hospital design and administration and could have been a huge failure. Instead, however, the facility soon became the best-known and perhaps the most well respected hospital in the Confederacy. Its success made it an obvious model to follow and prompted the adoption of the pavilion style and organizational structure wherever possible throughout the Confederacy.

CHAPTER 2

Dr. James Brown McCaw
and the Surgeons

The operation of Chimborazo Hospital was an enormous task that required hundreds of people working in various positions. The 1862 army medical regulations allowed a hospital one medical officer for seventy patients, one nurse for every ten patients, one laundress for every twenty patients, and one cook for every thirty patients.[1] Since each of Chimborazo's five division hospitals averaged a patient census of approximately 600, the number of hospital attendants allowed was 60 nurses, 30 laundresses, and 20 cooks per hospital—or 550 attendants at Chimborazo. The numbers do not include the matrons or any of the support staff who served in miscellaneous positions. Although Chimborazo's staff never reached the number of workers allowed because of shortages of competent workers, the numbers illustrate the magnitude of the hospital. An article in *The Richmond Examiner* reported 45 medical staff, 45 matrons, and 120 support staff at Chimborazo.[2]

The people who staffed the hospital represented all levels of Southern society: wealthy white men as surgeons, middle-class merchants as apothecaries, skilled workers as blacksmiths and carpenters, farmers and common workers as detailed enlisted men, respectable ladies as matrons, and free blacks and hired slaves as nurses, laundresses, and cooks. To keep the various people working together smoothly required organization and careful management. For maximum efficiency, the staff was organized on a hierarchical model based on a military chain of command. The senior medical officers filled the top level, followed by the junior officers, then the detailed enlisted men, with the free blacks and slaves at Chimborazo on the bottom level. The positions of non-military workers who did not fit into the above categories were often determined by their skills and usefulness as much as by the hospital's policy. The definition of the duties of each hospital position was standardized as much as possible by the Surgeon General's Office and printed in a yearly edition of the army's medical regulations.

One position, however, that medical regulations did not address was that of the chief administrator of large multi-hospitals such as Chimborazo. These administrators, referred to as surgeons-in-chief, held unique positions that went far beyond the duties of surgeon or even surgeon-in-charge. James Brown McCaw, the chief administrator at Chimborazo, was the first Confederate surgeon to hold such a position. Never before in American history had a physician been placed in charge of such a large hospital, military or civilian. McCaw's interpretation of this new position would have long-term effects on not only his hospital but also the Confederate medical system. The quick success of Chimborazo convinced Surgeon General Moore of the merit of large hospital complexes with a surgeon-in-chief as the administrative head of the facility. The success of Chimborazo made it the pattern on which many other Confederate hospitals were formed. McCaw's actions as the first surgeon-in-chief set precedents that directly affected all five of the multi-hospitals in the Richmond area. Thus, McCaw's influence was not limited only to the administration of his hospital, which served almost eighty thousand patients, but also spread to the other multi-hospitals and large general hospitals in Virginia that provided medical care for the majority of the Confederacy's wounded.

Before the war, civilian hospitals were managed by a superintendent and a board of trustees. The main qualifications for a superintendent were good character and thriftiness. Superintendents received little training in hospital management since the trustees oversaw all major decisions. Physicians generally had little voice in the hospital's daily operations. McCaw did not run his hospital according to this pattern. He used the military nature of his facility to provide an organizational hierarchy and discipline. He had no board of trustees to which he had to answer. His superiors were happy as long as he could provide good patient care and follow the regulations of the Medical Department. As a physician he could implement policies that focused on patient care and sound medical practice. McCaw did not limit himself to the challenges of administrator and physician. He realized the importance of public opinion and worked to make his facility accessible to visitors who would tell others of the positive things going on at his hospital. He did not promote his hospital to get patients, of which he had a guaranteed, constant supply; rather, he realized that he could improve the morale of the patients and the public by showing them that the soldiers were being well cared for in the hospitals. While trying to accomplish the tasks he set for himself, he redefined hospital management.

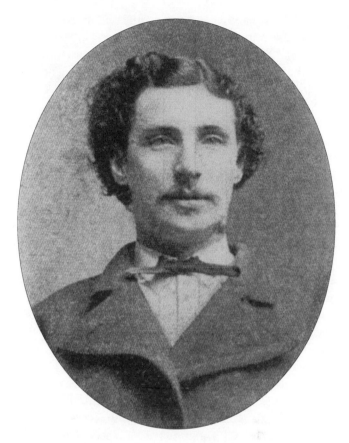

James Brown McCaw, c. 1850. Print courtesy of the
Museum of the Confederacy, Richmond, Virginia.

Surgeon General Moore's decision to form such a large institution as Chimborazo required him to find the right individual to lead it. We do not know specifically why he chose McCaw, but the well-known and respected Richmond physician and professor does seem to have been a good choice. Physically, McCaw was a commanding figure described as "a well-built man with a contained, strongly designed face and resolute eyes."[3]

McCaw was the fourth generation in his family to be a physician and the third generation to practice in Richmond.[4] After attending the Richmond Academy for his early education, McCaw traveled to New York to study at the Medical College of the University of New York under Dr. Valentine Mott, a world-renowned surgeon.[5] The Medical College had been founded in 1839 and typically provided an ungraded two-year program for its students. The institution's goal, "the building up [of] a national school worthy of the country and the age," prompted it to purchase an expensive "Chemical and Philosophical Apparatus of the best description." The medical school was close to hospitals and dispensaries and encouraged (but did not require) clinical work of its students.[6] In March 1844 James McCaw graduated from the school with his degree in medicine from the University of New York. After living for a brief time in Charles City County, he returned to Richmond to build up his practice. In 1845 he married Delia Patteson of Richmond.[7]

Over the next fifteen years, McCaw's reputation as a trusted physician steadily grew. Besides working as a general practitioner with a focus on the diseases of women and children, McCaw began to expand his sphere of influence. He was a member of the Medical Society of Virginia and once president of the Richmond Academy of Medicine. In the 1850s he also held key editorial positions for several Virginia medical journals. From 1854 to 1855 he served as the editor of the *Virginia Medical and Surgical Journal*, and from January 1856 to December 1859, he was the co-editor of the *Virginia Medical Journal*.[8] The *Virginia Medical Journal*, which declared itself "unconnected with any local institution or association," was designed to be "the independent advocate of the rights and interests of the entire medical public." The journal, published twice a year, included lithographs and wood engravings along with approximately eleven hundred pages of text.[9] In 1860 this journal's name was changed to the *Maryland and Virginia Medical Journal*; its last volume was printed in 1861.

The connections McCaw made through his work with the journals are notable. Dr. George Alexander Otis (1830–1881) worked with McCaw as a co-editor and a corresponding editor in 1854. During the war, Otis served as a surgeon for a regiment from Massachusetts (his home state) before being transferred to the U.S. Army Surgeon General's Office and given the task of collecting materialsfor a surgical history of the war. Later, as the curator of the Army Medical Museum, he edited the surgical volumes of *The Medical and Surgical History of the War of the Rebellion*.[10] Another prominent figure, Dr. William Alexander Hammond of Maryland, worked with McCaw as a co-editor for the *Maryland and Virginia Medical Journal*.

In 1858 Dr. McCaw became a professor of chemistry and pharmacy at the Medical College of Virginia. His connection with the medical school, the only one open in the South during the Civil War, continued throughout the war.[11] His position at the college, as editor of medical journals, and as a leader in Richmond's medical community made him aware of new medical treatments and innovative approaches to medicine and made him an obvious choice to command the new hospital.

Perhaps the reasons for McCaw's appointment and success as the director of Chimborazo Hospital went beyond his medical knowledge and included his personal demeanor. The *Dictionary of American Biography* describes McCaw as "a man of striking presence and forceful but genial personality."[12] A sense of how McCaw's personal demeanor affected his work at Chimborazo was provided by a description of the surgeon in the journal of Phoebe Yates Pember, the head matron at Chimborazo No. 2:

> He was energetic—capable—skillful. A man with ready oil to pour upon troubled waters. Difficulties melted away beneath the warmth of his ready interest, and mountains sank into mole-hills when his quick comprehension had surmounted and leveled them. However troublesome daily increasing annoyances became, if they could not be removed, his few and ready words sent applicants and grumblers home satisfied to do the best they could.[13]

Ernest Furgurson wrote a similar description of McCaw in his book on Confederate Richmond: "He was an ingenious administrator who got his way with gentlemanly persuasion rather than martial bluster."[14] After a thorough examination of the sources on Chimborazo and McCaw, the impression one gets of McCaw is that of a remarkable Southern gentleman: a man of integrity who was a good judge of people, who cared about his staff and patients, and who tempered his requests and orders with wisdom and humor.

McCaw's varied accomplishments were impressive. His most obvious fault was not following the details of medical regulations with regard to reports and the limits of the hospital fund as closely as Moore would have liked. However, even this fault can be easily excused when seen in the light of McCaw's focus on patient care. Reports could wait if it meant helping patients. The regulations limiting the use of the hospital fund could be stretched to provide better supplies for his hospital. Chimborazo Hospital was fortunate to have the leadership of McCaw, just as McCaw was fortunate to have the support and respect of Surgeon General Moore and Medical Director William Carrington. Throughout the Union and Confederacy, there were many other examples of fine physicians who were allowed to develop their potential as surgeons and administrators for the good of their patients and the cause.

One such example, Samuel H. Stout, rose quickly through the Confederate Medical Department from a surgeon to a post surgeon and finally to the medical director of hospitals for the Army of Tennessee. Stout's position was unique in the Confederacy; he oversaw over sixty hospitals located from Montgomery, Alabama, to Augusta, Georgia. In her biography of Stout, Glenna Schroeder-Lein praised his ability as a talented administrator.[15]

Perhaps the most notable figure in the Union Medical Department was William Alexander Hammond, who had probably met McCaw when both were medical students in New York. Hammond's preceptor, William Holme Van Buren, was the son-in-law and protégé of Valentine Mott, under whom McCaw had studied. Hammond came to New York to study the year McCaw graduated.[16] After gaining clinical experience in Philadelphia and New York hospitals, Hammond served as an assistant surgeon for the U.S. Army from 1849 until 1860, when he left the army to teach anatomy and physiology at the University of Maryland Medical School. When the war broke out, he reenlisted. Then only thirty-three years old, the tall, stout, confident physician petitioned for a suspension of the thirty-five-year-old age requirement so that he could receive a surgeon's rank.

As an assistant surgeon, he organized several military hospitals in Maryland and Pennsylvania. According to his biographer, Bonnie Ellen Blustein, "Hammond threw himself into [his] work with energy and impatience. . . . [H]e inaugurated the employment of civilian cooks and female nurses . . . a fairly innovative plan. . . . He requisitioned additional buildings and medical cadets to help staff them. He personally attended to such details as the purchase of mattresses and comforters and the acquisition of a supply of smallpox vaccine."[17] After only seven months he became a medical purveyor, then received a promotion to inspector of hospitals two months later in March 1862. As an inspector he reported on the horrible conditions he found and recommended replacing the existing buildings with "a series of 'huts' capable of holding fifty patients each. These would be arranged in 'echelons' to allow proper ventilation."[18] This plan, of course, was remarkably similar to how Chimborazo had been constructed. It is unknown whether Hammond and McCaw took this idea from their shared medical education or developed it during the 1850s when they worked together as editors.

In April 1862, with the support of the United States Sanitary Commission, Hammond became the new surgeon general of the U.S. medical department. While in this position he revealed ideas about hospital construction and administration very similar to those of McCaw. Blustein wrote:

> One of Hammond's first pet projects was the construction of a model hospital in West Philadelphia. He 'draughted the plans, had a supervision of its construction, and personally selected its corps of physicians.' The facilities originally consisted of 'twenty-one one-story buildings, arranged in the form of a parallelogram.' . . . [T]here was to be one responsible medical officer in charge of each building. Unlike civilian hospitals, there would be no lay board of managers to meddle in his affairs. . . . Hammond emphasized that the steward assigned to each hospital would be subordinate to all the medical officers. This hospital would be controlled by physicians; it would be a medical, not a charity, institution.[19]

Hammond's hospital encountered severe problems, ranging from shortages of civilian staffing to difficulties in getting patients.

As surgeon general, Hammond worked to organize all the North's resources into a national military hospital system and successfully met many challenges. He sponsored the hiring of female nurses to alleviate the shortage in hospitals, advocated the designation of special wards within larger hospitals for certain illnesses, and placed medical books and clinical medical instruments on the army medical supply table. "His creative imagination and ineradicable curiosity," noted Blustein, "were among his greatest personal assets, but he lacked both patience and 'inflexibility of purpose.'"[20] His assertive manner and dogmatic determination ruffled too many feathers in the hot political environment and resulted in his removal as surgeon general after only eighteen months in the position.[21]

While Hammond was busy reorganizing the Union medical department, McCaw worked to hammer out the details of the model hospital that he and Hammond evidently shared. The most challenging aspect was to do so while learning what medical regulations did and did not allow him to do. On numerous occasions during the first few years of the war, Moore wrote to McCaw to explain that something he did was not allowed by regulations. One early example concerned leaves of absence. On December 30, 1861, Moore wrote, "It having been reported to this Office by the Inspector of Hospitals that Leaves of Absence are granted the Medical Officers of your Hospital by your authority: I have to inform you that such authority is not recognized by the Army Regulations."[22] Slowly but surely, McCaw figured out the boundaries of his authority and the military bureaucracy and, while doing so, successfully organized the Chimborazo complex.

Overall, the challenge of being an effective surgeon-in-chief required organization, flexibility, and creativity. Glenna Schroeder-Lein stated well the talents needed to be an effective hospital administrator in her biography of Samuel Stout: "It was a rare doctor who had the administrative skills, perhaps even genius, to put all aspects of a hospital together: to learn how to adapt to military regulations, how to use the hospital fund to the best advantage, how to keep a hospital clean, and how to discipline and supervise subordinates and patients without causing a mutiny."[23]

McCaw's personality and management style are important to understand, since all large organizations commonly reflect the temperament of their leadership. As he developed his hospital and his administrative position, McCaw made his decisions based on the concept of what best improved patient care. He recognized that his main job was not to keep personalities happy or the bureaucracy running smoothly but to see that his hospital provided the best patient care available. Whenever a hospital administrator manages his facility with that approach, all of the people who work and stay at that hospital can discern it. If a difficulty arises, there is a confidence permeating the hospital environment that the problem will be solved. Throughout the war McCaw ably kept his focus on patient care and learned how to use the authority and bureaucracy of the military to provide for the needs of his patients and staff. He also understood the importance of the perception that the people of the Confederacy had of his hospital.

An important feature of the focus on patient care involved McCaw's understanding of the importance of morale and mental health to promoting physical health. "Paying great attention to diet," wrote Clifford Dowdey, "he used sunlight and fresh air and space for mental therapy and created an atmosphere more of barracks than a retreat for the sick."[24] Perhaps his years of practice as a women's and children's physician contributed to his awareness of the mind-body connection.

Administrative duties filled much of McCaw's time. His official duties included supervising the five hospitals at Chimborazo and their medical officers, relaying any official orders for the post, maintaining communications with the surgeon general and medical director, and filling out the many reports required by the Confederate Medical Department. McCaw's office was responsible each day for collecting the morning reports from each of the hospital's five divisions; they then sent a copy of Chimborazo's consolidated morning report and a transcript of all admissions and discharges to Moore's office. Reports required weekly or monthly included a statement of the hospital fund, reports of surgical cases, and reports showing the detail or return of medical officers, hospital staff, and patients. As the war continued, the required reports became more numerous and more complex; printed forms, provided by the Medical Department, helped to ease the clerks' load as this happened.[25] Copies of all reports, as well as current lists of Chimborazo's employees and accounts of hospital property, were also kept in the main office. During 1861 and 1862, McCaw addressed any questions he might have to the Surgeon General's Office. Starting in January 1863, William Carrington, serving as the medical director of Virginia, received most of McCaw's correspondence. A number of clerks helped McCaw fill out and copy the appropriate reports and perform the other necessary record keeping. Chimborazo's central office, located in the two-story house on the hospital's grounds, stayed busy coordinating activities between the different hospitals, departments, and offices at Chimborazo.

McCaw's office also arranged for the transfer of patients to and from Chimborazo. The earliest surviving transfer order was dated January 7, 1862. The order requested that two hundred patients "who have been slightly wounded, and who have not been exposed directly to the contagion of Smallpox" be sent to the general hospital at Danville.[26] Ambulances brought patients to the hospital's central office, where they registered and waited to be distributed to a division. A clerk recorded each patient's name, rank, regiment, and company into the central register. This register kept track of which of the hospital's divisions the patient was assigned to so that mail, pay, and supplies could be properly routed. When the patient left Chimborazo, the main office recorded the date and destination at the time of his departure.

While his office took care of most of the record keeping and general reports, McCaw's attention went mainly to the management of the people who lived and worked at the hospital and to the management of the hospital fund. Choosing Chimborazo's personnel was one part of McCaw's job. Although surgeons and other medical officers were assigned to Chimborazo's various hospitals, it is likely that McCaw had some input as to which medical officers received assignments to his hospital. Several physicians wrote to him, seeking to serve at his hospital. In July 1862 a contract surgeon wrote of his service at Manassas and other battles near Richmond, asking to be hired at Chimborazo. Earlier the same month, a field surgeon requested that McCaw intervene on his behalf with the surgeon general so that he could be transferred to Chimborazo; evidently, this man had made the same request of McCaw previously. McCaw wrote back, politely telling him that he should serve some time in the field first.[27] These requests and denials suggest that McCaw was unwilling to allow anyone to be part of his medical staff unless he was certain of that person's medical skill. It is possible that McCaw's influence over assignments of medical staff extended even beyond Chimborazo. In 1863 N. J. Walker sent a letter of introduction to McCaw for Dr. Saul Boyle, a physician on his way to Richmond to volunteer as a surgeon for the Confederacy. Walker stated, "Any facility which you may be able to afford Dr. Boyle in obtaining a position where he can be useful to our suffering troops will be most highly appreciated by him."[28]

McCaw also hired all other hospital personnel, from chief matrons to the slaves working in the laundries. The records reveal letters that McCaw received from prospective matrons, stewards, and clerks, in addition to numerous letters of recommendation for those individuals seeking employment at Chimborazo. Because Chimborazo was usually understaffed, McCaw had to allocate his workers carefully to ensure a working balance between the numbers of patients and caretakers in each hospital. Even though his hospitals were understaffed, however, McCaw realized that problem employees were not worth the trouble they caused. On several occasions he refused to have certain employees work at Chimborazo. A good example was a matron under Phoebe Pember's supervision in hospital No. 2 who was sent away by Pember after the woman caused numerous problems. McCaw supported Pember, and although the woman enlisted the sympathy of Medical Director Carrington, McCaw held his ground and refused to allow her to return.[29]

McCaw also attempted to help his employees with their workload. He did not want the patients in his hospitals to suffer from lack of care nor did he want his staff to be overworked, which would eventually affect patient care. When Chimborazo's census rose to record levels in 1863, McCaw continued to hire workers to meet the demand, even though his opinion of the numbers necessary significantly exceeded what medical regulations allowed. When Medical Department officials realized the discrepancy, they wrote to McCaw: "The number of attendants and employees is greatly beyond the proportion allowed by . . . Medical Regulations. . . . You are, therefore, directed immediately to reduce the number of attendants to accord with . . . Regulations, and to repost the excess to this office for final disposition."[30]

McCaw delegated a great deal of authority to his medical officers and the matrons, but he also kept a careful eye on the activities of the hospital. He inspected the hospitals daily and talked with the physicians and staff he encountered about their activities and concerns. Those daily walks allowed him to keep his finger on the pulse of Chimborazo and helped to maintain the morale of co-workers, many of whom looked to him when problems arose. Pember remembered, "[Dr. McCaw] was an unfailing refuge in times of distress, and whenever broken down by fatigue and small miseries I sought his advise [sic] and assistance, the first was not only the very best that could be secured, but unlike most of its kind, palatable; and the last entirely efficient."[31]

Moreover, the departments at Chimborazo that served all five of its hospitals, such as the guardhouse, bakery, and canal boat, reported directly to McCaw. Several notes survive in Chimborazo's records from guards asking McCaw for instructions whenever unusual matters arose. On one occasion, B. H. Huestis, the sergeant commander of the guard, reported that on the previous night at about nine o'clock he had arrested "two men of Suspicious Character they were Both asleep near the Bath House when found." Huestis asked, "What disposition shall I make of them?"[32]

As commandant, McCaw was also the highest judge at Chimborazo. He mediated any problems that arose between surgeons-in-charge or between managers in different parts of the Chimborazo complex. I. N. Fauit, the person in charge of the deadhouse of Division No. 5, wrote to McCaw of two bodies, "One entirely naked and the other with only a pair of pants." He requested help so that the men could "be properly dressed before burial." McCaw drafted a quick note to Dr. Seabrook, the surgeon-in-charge of No. 5, ordering him to take care of it.[33] Also, McCaw made himself available to Chimborazo's employees if an unsolvable dispute arose between them and their supervisors. Pember considered McCaw a good judge. She wrote, "No one ever applied to him in vain for either justice or courtesy."[34]

The judicious administration of the hospital fund was another of McCaw's key duties. When a soldier was admitted to a hospital, the value of his rations went into the hospital fund. The value of any items obtained by that hospital from the Commissary Department was subtracted from the fund, using contract or cost prices. The surgeon-in-charge, or surgeon-in-chief at the large hospitals, used the fund by authorizing the purchase of food and supplies not obtainable through government channels. Because food items issued to regular soldiers were often not appropriate for soldiers in a hospital, medical regulations allowed the hospital fund to be used "in the purchase of any article for the subsistence or comfort of the sick, not authorized to be otherwise furnished."[35] The judicious use of the hospital fund frequently made the difference between a well-supplied hospital and a poorly supplied one. The fund and its proper use baffled many surgeons, especially in the early years of the war. According to Glenna Schroeder-Lein, Samuel Stout "speculated that as much as one million dollars was lost and much needless suffering resulted during the early part of the war because of lack of knowledge about this money."[36] McCaw quickly learned not only how to use this fund but how to do so creatively. In addition to its obvious uses, he utilized the fund to purchase a canal boat to transport supplies, hired agents to negotiate the best prices for rare items, and made other improvements to the hospital's physical and manpower resources.

Another feature of McCaw's position was maintaining communications between his facility and the outside world. In Chimborazo's records are numerous examples of the many types of letters McCaw received and responded to. Most of the surviving letters were from Moore or Carrington, requesting information or issuing orders. Other official correspondence included mundane requests from different groups in the army that dealt with the hospital. Some examples exist, however, that illustrate how McCaw's concern for patient care and good medicine prompted him to take action even when the matter did not involve his hospital. He wrote one letter to the medical director, admonishing the physicians at Richmond's Receiving Hospital for their faulty diagnoses of patients then sent to Chimborazo. After the medical director questioned W. J. Coffur, the surgeon-in-charge of the receiving hospital about the matter, Coffur wrote to McCaw, at "the earliest opportunity," informing him that "the evil spoken of is corrected here as far as practicable." He explained, "[T]he very short time in which the patient is allowed to remain makes it impracticable to arrive at an accurate diagnosis in many cases— The Hospital discovering the fault can very easily return the men to duty."[37]

Not all of McCaw's correspondence came from an official source, however. In fact, numerous examples survive of letters from individuals who needed information of some kind from him. An article in a Richmond newspaper informed interested citizens that "Letters addressed to Box 542 will be distributed daily from the Hospital P.O. & all persons seeking information on any subject appertaining to the Institution, or with regard to any of its inmates will receive a prompt response by address of JB McCaw, Senior Surgeon, Chimborazo Hospital."[38] Although responding to these letters could become tedious, McCaw realized how important it was for the perception of the hospital to be positive. One way to do this was to make information available to those whose friends and relatives were patients there.

McCaw received numerous letters concerning individual patients. One letter, dated April 3, 1862, was from General Benjamin W. S. Cabell concerning the death of his son and the disposition of his son's belongings:

I beg respectfully to ask you, Sir, Why was I not informed of my son's arrival at the Hospital when he first got there? Why was not my numerous friends and relations informed of the fact? . . . any one of them would have received, and treated him with all possible affection and kindness—all of them, not more than two miles distant? Why not inform the family, of every one, whether the humble or the enabled, when their relations get there?[39]

McCaw's response, dated April 5, attempted to explain the situation: "We received in March 2900 patients and it is easy to see that . . . It is simply impossible to inform the families of 2900 men (coming from Maryland to Texas) what time their relations reached the hospital."[40] Another example of this type of correspondence was a request from William Clopton, evidently a friend of McCaw, who wrote asking that his son be furloughed from Chimborazo. McCaw declined, writing, "Pvt Wm Clopton is not very sick. I think he will be able to return to his Regt in ten or twelve days."[41]

Numerous charity groups also wrote to Chimborazo Hospital, asking for information about what the soldiers needed or voicing concerns about whether their donated goods had been received. F. W. Bridgeforth of Lumberg, Virginia, wrote concerning "the box [of provisions], barrel of potatoes, coop of chickens & firkin of butter" that his group had sent to the hospital. Bridgeforth had spoken to a wounded soldier who had been at Chimborazo who had told him that "those who most needed [the] delicacies seldom get them . . . and very frequently the delicacies intended for the sick are eaten, by fat sleek nurses, before the very eyes of the sick man." These remarks disturbed Bridgeforth: "Mine is a feeble voice to 'croak,' but these are wrongs that should be righted and that speedily."[42]

Even newspaper reporters contacted McCaw for information. In 1864 a reporter named E. E. Coerall asked that McCaw furnish him with a report of the number of sick and wounded at Chimborazo; Coerall, in turn, wanted to publish these figures in his paper. After receiving no response, Coerall wrote to McCaw:

I very much regret not receiving a report of sick and wounded remaining in your hospital per request, which I desired for publication. I had hoped, Sir, that your name would appear in newspaper with those of your . . . surgeons, and that an equally favorable report would be given. . . .
Having denied me the priviledge [sic] of receiving your report before I left Richmond, I trust you will forward it to Montgomery as early as practicable. Winder, Jackson and Howard's Grove have furnished their reports.[43]

McCaw wrote Carrington: "Res[ponse] referred to Med Director. Who is this man?" Carrington answered, "He is a reporter for a small paper in the south [the *Argus and*

Crisis]. The Surg Genl and the Supt A & O seem to think the desired publication will convey too much information to the enemy, and hence forbide the publication of these reports."[44] If Coerall had indeed received reports from Winder and the other hospitals, this matter could reveal a case of better judgment on the part of McCaw than that of other surgeons-in-chief.

Some of the letters McCaw received did not even refer to medicine or his work at Chimborazo but illustrate the reputation that McCaw had achieved throughout the South. An example of this type of miscellaneous correspondence came from Colonel Joel R. Griffin. Griffin explained that he wanted to establish a sugar refinery in western Georgia and requested "a complete Analysis of Sorghum Syrup so that I may the more systematically produce the Sugar." McCaw had been recommended to him "as a gentleman of large experience and fine Scientific attainment and as being one fully able to give . . . the analysis so much desired." There is no record of a reply from McCaw.[45]

In addition to his administrative responsibilities, McCaw acted as a surgeon for Chimborazo's Division No. 1. His military duties outside of Chimborazo included serving on the Executive Committee of the Confederate Medical Department and several boards of examiners.[46] Beyond his military obligations, McCaw continued to teach chemistry and pharmacy at the Medical College of Virginia and served as the main editor of the fourteen issues of the *Confederate States Medical and Surgical Journal*.

Underneath McCaw in Chimborazo's hierarchy were the surgeons-in-charge (also called division surgeons) of each of its five hospitals. Dr. P. F. Browne of Accomac, Virginia, was in charge of Chimborazo No. 1. In July 1861 Browne had joined the 39th Virginia regiment, with which he served until coming to Chimborazo in October. Dr. Stephen E. Habersham of Savannah, Georgia, was in charge of Chimborazo No. 2—his initial assignment after receiving his commission. Dr. Edwin Harvey Smith received his commission and was placed in charge of Chimborazo No. 3 in October 1861. Dr. William A. Davis was in charge of Chimborazo No. 4 from its opening in November 1861 to March 1865, when he left Chimborazo to become the medical purveyor for the Lynchburg area. Dr. E. M. Seabrook from Charleston, South Carolina, managed Chimborazo No. 5. Except for Davis's absence at the very end of the war, all five surgeons-in-charge of Chimborazo's divisions remained in their positions throughout the war, adding to the stability and effectiveness of the hospital. Their only recorded absences were for short periods during which they helped start other hospitals or served with the Reserve Surgical Corps in 1864.[47]

The major medical responsibilities of the surgeons-in-charge were of a supervisory nature. According to a circular from the Surgeon General's Office, surgeons-in-charge were expected to "act in the capacity of consulting physicians—giving to the junior Medical Officers in attendance the benefit of their more mature

---

TABLE 2
Surgeons-in-Charge at Chimborazo's Five Divisions

Hospital	Surgeon-in-Charge
Chimborazo No. 1	P. F. Browne
Chimborazo No. 2	Stephen E. Habersham
Chimborazo No. 3	Edwin Harvey Smith
Chimborazo No. 4	William A. Davis
Chimborazo No. 5	E. M. Seabrook

---

judgment and experience."[48] Pember described their duties as follows: "The surgeon in charge is always on the ground, goes through the wards daily, consulting with his assistants and reforming abuses."[49] In addition to their other medical duties, the surgeons-in-charge comprised the examining board at Chimborazo that determined which patients would be fit for duty in ten days, which could be transferred to private quarters, which could receive furloughs, and which would be discharged.[50] These surgeons were also responsible for the weekly examinations of any patients in private quarters.

In addition to his medical duties, the surgeon-in-charge of a hospital was responsible for ensuring that his division ran smoothly and effectively in its efforts to treat its sick and wounded patients. All the buildings and patients in his division were ultimately his responsibility. All outside orders came through McCaw for disbursement and enforcement. The surgeons-in-charge decided the ward assignments for incoming patients. The assistant surgeons and acting assistant surgeons, hospital stewards, and chief matron reported directly to the surgeon-in-charge with any questions or problems. Daily, the surgeon-in-charge furnished McCaw's office with a morning report for his division; inspected the wards, kitchens, and laundries under his command; and appointed one physician to serve as the division's officer of the day. Monthly, he filled out the required reports and approved the division's pay rolls. He also approved all requisitions for supplies beyond the hospital's grounds before they were sent to Chimborazo's central office.

Under the surgeons-in-charge were the rest of Chimborazo's physicians, who were classified as surgeons, assistant surgeons, and acting assistant surgeons. All surgeons held the rank of major, were at least twenty-five years old, had usually practiced medicine for at least five years, and had an established reputation within the medical community.[51] In October 1861 surgeons were paid a maximum of $200 per month for their services, in addition to allowances for quarters, fuel, and forage for their horses.[52]

Because of the high demand in the Confederate army for experienced physicians, Chimborazo had only six surgeons on its staff: McCaw and the five surgeons-in-chief. Most of the medical officers at Chimborazo were assistant surgeons. Assistant surgeons, who were generally between twenty-one and twenty-five years old, held the rank of captain and in October 1861 received a maximum salary of $150 per month.

To supplement the number of available medical officers at Chimborazo and other hospitals, the medical director hired "contract physicians." The Medical Department designated these physicians acting assistant surgeons and gave them the temporary rank of second lieutenant. The contract physicians agreed to conform to the army's Medical Department regulations and perform the normal duties of a medical officer, except for accompanying troops on marches or transports. They received eighty dollars per month for their services in October 1861—about half the salary of an assistant surgeon.[53] The negotiated amount could be slightly higher. It normally depended on whether "he [was] required to abandon his own business, and give his whole time to the public service."[54] Although few distinctions seem to have been made on an everyday basis between regular medical officers and contract surgeons, there were some distinctions. Perhaps the most visible was that contract surgeons were not allowed to wear the medical corps uniform, although the distinction might not have been critically important since few medical officers wore the regulation uniforms on a daily basis.[55]

In some cases civilian physicians offered their services to the Confederate Medical Department free of charge during emergency situations. Medical Director Carrington wrote Dr. McCaw about Dr. Knox, a Richmond physician, who had offered to do this. Knox was temporarily assigned to ward duty at Chimborazo, although he was not able to serve as officer of the day.[56]

The surgeon-in-charge of the hospital assigned the assistant surgeons and acting assistant surgeons from one to three wards. Two full wards with forty patients each would give one doctor the responsibility for eighty patients. At times, even during a period of average census, the ratio of patients to physicians would grow even larger when a physician became ill or when physicians were away on leave or on temporary duty in the field or at other hospitals. As P. F. Browne, the surgeon-in-charge of Chimborazo No. 1, told McCaw on June 18, 1863: "Two of my Asst Surgeons are sick, which leaves only three on duty. I have a population today of nearly four hundred men with a large portion of sick and wounded soldiers. I respectfully ask that you send me, without delay, an intelligent and reliable Asst Surgeon."[57] Thus, the patient-doctor ratio of that division was more than 133 to 1. Medical Director Carrington, who had received the letter forwarded by McCaw, returned one assistant surgeon to Chimborazo whom he had reassigned the day before and advised a shifting of medical officers among the divisions to compensate for the shortage at Chimborazo No. 1. According to Carrington's reply, with the new officer, the 33 medical officers at Chimborazo's hospitals should be able to care for the 1,500 patients there.[58] The corresponding ratio computes to just over 45 patients for each physician.

When a new patient was admitted to a ward, the doctor responsible for that ward examined him, writing the diagnosis and the appropriate diet for that patient on the paper ticket kept at the end of the bed. The doctors made rounds at least twice a day, usually in the morning and afternoon, at which time they gave instructions to the nurses regarding the patients' care and prescribed the appropriate medications. Each day at noon, the ward physicians met with their surgeon-in-charge to inform him of the condition of their patients, as well as to report any neglect of duty by their ward masters or nurses. Assistant surgeons were expected to stay on Chimborazo's grounds throughout the day.[59]

When necessary, medical officers were given additional duties. In addition to being responsible for the tent wards of Chimborazo No. 4, Dr. W. C. Kloman was assigned by Surgeon-in-Charge Davis upon the request of McCaw to visit the guardhouse daily to attend to any sick there.[60] Surgeons and assistant surgeons could also be assigned to temporary duty in the field or to other hospitals. The surgeons were typically chosen by the medical director, while McCaw usually made the decisions involving his assistant surgeons' assignments.

Some of the physicians at Chimborazo and other Richmond hospitals served in the Reserve Surgical Corps during the last years of the war. This corps was used to supplement the number of medical officers available to care for the wounded in field hospitals at battle sites that were not too far from the surgeons' permanent assignments. A purveying officer accompanied the corps and provided the necessary medicines and dressings. The biggest obstacle to overcome for surgeons who wanted this experience was obtaining a set of surgical instruments that they could take with them to the battlefield.[61]

Assistant surgeons and acting assistant surgeons were also required to serve as the officer of the day on a rotating basis. The duties of this position lasted for a twenty-four hour period, beginning at 10:00 A.M., and required, among other things, that the physician remain at his division throughout the day and night and oversee the handling of the bodies of any patients who died. As S. E. Habersham, the surgeon-in-charge of Chimbarazo No. 2, told the assistant surgeons under him: "[The officer] will see that the body is properly prepared and certainly dead before being sent to the dead house."[62] The officer of the day also double-checked the ticket placed on the body and the notation recorded in the dead book.

Another duty of the officer of the day was to inspect all his hospital's buildings and make a written report of his inspection and the day's events to his surgeon-in-charge. The complexity of these reports varied from one doctor to another. Many officers wrote only enough to show that they had indeed inspected the hospital as they should. E. W. Gordon, an assistant surgeon, provided a typical example of this type of report after serving as officer of the day for Chimborazo No. 2 on December 8, 1864: "I report the wards, kitchen & premisis [*sic*] of this Division in usual condition: tolerably good. The *Privy* needs cleaning & scouring."[63] Other officers wrote detailed reports that thoroughly addressed the situation of their hospital that day.

When the condition of a patient required it, the ward physicians sometimes spent the night in the wards. More commonly, only the officer of the day slept at the hospital, leaving the other officers free to return to their homes or boarding houses in the city. If they chose to room away from the hospital, they received a commutation for quarters from the quartermaster's department. Physicians who lived at the hospital were provided fuel and stabling; those drawing commutation were not allowed to use the hospital's stables or fuel. In March 1862 there were accommodations for twelve assistant surgeons at Chimborazo, with plans to build more if needed.[64] Toward the end of the war, Chimborazo's assistant surgeons learned of a plan to quarter them in vacated patient wards at their hospital, thus ridding the government of the expense of paying any expenses for accommodations outside hospital grounds. In response, they appealed in writing to the surgeon general not to implement his plan: "The wards of this hospital being hastily and imperfectly constructed would require a thorough remodeling or even an entire rebuilding 'de novo' to render them tenable during the coming winter. In the construction of Officers Quarters . . . some regard has been had to the comfort of the occupants."[65] Whether the officers' petition succeeded is questionable. In November 1864 several medical officers complained of the conditions of the officers' sleeping room in reports to their surgeon-in-charge. E. W. Gordon wrote, "The officers' sleeping room is quite open & uncomfortable during the night."[66] Surgeons were allowed to reside with their families in Richmond throughout the war.

Many horror stories can be found in Civil War literature about the quality of physicians in this era. This is not surprising since the public had a low level of respect for physicians in general. Physicians in antebellum America lacked the major characteristics of a successful profession. Much medical education was insufficient, requiring only ten months of lectures and lacking practical training or experience in a clinical setting. Medical licensing laws had collapsed in the early 1830s because of the disorganization within the medical community, which decreased requirements to obtain a license, and the difficulty of enforcing existing licensing laws. "[T]he practice of medicine," according to Martin Kaufman, "was open to anyone who considered himself qualified."[67] The American public preferred a physician to have a degree from a medical school, but because of the decreasing quality of medical education, a diploma did not guarantee medical knowledge. Faced with a wide variety of physicians and having little means to ensure the skill of a physician, the public normally depended on their personal experiences and the opinions of friends and family to evaluate a doctor's knowledge and abilities. During the war, patients had no choice regarding their physician—they knew nothing about the man on whose skill their lives sometimes depended.

Some problems with physicians and medical care were almost certain when, early in the war, civilian physicians were suddenly placed within a military bureaucracy and asked to treat horrible battlefield wounds and uncommon illnesses. However, as medical historian H. H. Cunningham noted, one astute Confederate private "pointed out in the Summer of 1864 that it was 'usual to abuse doctors all over the world. . . . Complaints of hospital arrangements are consequently not infrequently unreasonable, and anathemas upon surgeons upon insufficient grounds.'"[68]

Common complaints focused on the apathy and neglect that some doctors exhibited toward their patients. The complaints quickly received the attention of Confederate officials. The Confederate Congress discussed the issue and set up several committees to investigate reported problems. The committees found few problems that seemed common among medical physicians or facilities but did their best to fix the problems they did discover. One issue addressed was complaints of drunkenness—a problem not limited to the medical corps, of course, but perhaps more pervasive there early in the war because of easy access to liquor. In 1862 the Congress put the liquor cabinets in hospitals under the control of its matrons. Overall, as Cunningham has explained, "For every case of proved neglect of disabled men by their medical officers may be cited numerous instances of such officers' devotion and self-sacrifice."[69] Cunningham concluded, "There can be no question, of course, but that some ignorant and incompetent practitioners found their way into the Confederate Medical Department. It is doubtful, however, that the percentage of undesirables was high."[70]

One major safeguard that the Confederate Medical Department utilized was a medical exam. "Whereas the Union army relied largely upon state-appointed regimental surgeons," noted John Duffy, "the Confederate government directly commissioned its approximately 5,800 medical officers. Medical examining boards interviewed all candidates from the beginning, thus keeping the number of incompetents to a minimum."[71] The medical examining boards consisted of at least three army surgeons and convened on a regular basis to review the applications of physicians who wanted to become surgeons or assistant surgeons. All candidates were required to practice orthodox medicine, which meant that no homeopathic or other medical-sect practitioners would be allowed in the medical corps. Medical regulations stated, "The board will scrutinize rigidly the moral habits, professional acquirements, and physical qualifications of the candidates, and report favorably, either for appointment or promotion, in no case admitting of a reasonable doubt."[72]

Good character was also seen as a critical element of a successful physician. Character could be judged by the general public, whereas few individuals were educated enough to be able to judge a physician's medical knowledge or competence. "As a speaker reminded the graduating class of medical students at Harvard in 1870," John Harley Warner noted, "their success in American society 'depended fully as much upon what they were as upon what they knew.'"[73] In a speech to the graduates of the University of Pennsylvania in 1841, George B. Wood explained another important reason for the emphasis on a physician's character: "He should have the graces of gentlemanly deportment and familiarity with the conventional forms of good breeding; so that he may avoid wounding the often morbid delicacy of his patients, and adding the irritations of an offended taste or ruffled temper to the evils of disease."[74]

In addition to a physician's personal demeanor and local reputation, nineteenth-century Americans also considered the person's level of education and charitable service to the community as ways to judge character. The idea of character was often associated with obtaining a liberal education. If a person had attended a university and had obtained a classical education, that person was seen as possessing some qualifications to practice medicine, even if he had not attended a medical school. Another means by which a physician could improve his status in the community was by conducting laboratory work in physiology or chemistry or being involved with another scientific pursuit. These scientific activities were viewed as an expression of cultural participation, not unlike leadership in civic groups such as museum societies.[75] Also, laboratory work suggested the physician's discipline and commitment to hard work—both good moral characteristics.

While an examining board measured the candidate's character mainly using letters of reference, it tested medical knowledge in a more direct manner. Both oral and written examinations were given to all candidates. If successful, an applicant would receive a commission as assistant surgeon within two years. If unsuccessful, the applicant might be allowed a second examination after a certain period. Early in the war applicants had to wait at least six months; by 1863 a two-year wait was implemented.[76] After two failures, no further examinations would be given to that applicant. The boards also examined assistant surgeons who wanted promotion to surgeon. Schroeder-Lein explained that a typical written exam for promotion was four pages long:

> [The forty-eight questions] asked the meaning of various terms, the proper dosages of various medications, the antidotes to certain poisons, the route of blood circulating from particular organs to the heart, the circumstances rendering amputation necessary, procedures for the treatment of gunshot wounds, and the nature, diagnosis, and treatment of particular diseases.[77]

If an applicant for promotion refused to take the examination or failed it, "he cease[d] to be a medical officer of the army."[78]

Medical examining boards did receive some criticism. The examinations were not standardized throughout the Confederacy, and undoubtedly some boards performed their duties better than others. However, all of the examiners did hold the rank of surgeon and did understand that an error in their judgment about a physician could be a matter of life or death for a number of Confederate soldiers. Even if the nature of specific questions on the exams varied, the presence of medical examinations as a prerequisite to become a medical officer helped to ensure the caliber of the Confederacy's medical officers. Statistics are not available to reveal the percentage of candidates who failed the exams, but the records do reveal that some were rejected. George E. Waller, a hospital steward who was examined unsuccessfully before the medical board in Richmond, explained the extent of his exam. The examiners began by questioning him on the eye, the brain, "the various distrabution [sic] of the nerves, the artaries [sic] with their distrabutions [sic] and ramifications," dislocations of the hip, pneumonia, "and a thousand other questions that I do not recolect [sic]. . . . And after all this, they gave me a sheet of Foolscap just as full of questions as it could be." Waller further stated, "I was not at all disappointed when I was pitched for I had talked with Peticolas prior to my examination and he told he that four out of five wer [sic] thrown."[79]

Contract physicians were not examined by medical boards as were regular medical officers. Schroeder-Lein explained that "[w]hile some of these doctors were well-qualified men awaiting an opportunity to appear before the examining board, others had failed the examinations or were physically unqualified for long-term service."[80] The practice of hiring physicians who had failed their medical boards was discontinued in December of 1863.[81]

After physicians passed their exams, the Surgeon General's Office took measures to ensure the quality of medical officers. To enhance the knowledge and skills of medical officers further, the Surgeon General's Office circulated numerous memos concerning the proper treatment of different injuries and illnesses, published Chisolm's *Manual of Military Surgery* in 1863, put medical textbooks and reference books on the supply table, and later in the war sponsored the creation and distribution of *The Confederate States Medical and Surgical Journal*. Also, reprimands were given for inappropriate behavior. Drunkenness was dealt with harshly. Samuel Stout reported, "Whenever I hear of a med. officer getting drunk, I notify him, that he must take his choice between a court-martial and resignation."[82] In September 1864 Moore instructed Carrington regarding one assistant surgeon's "dissapated habits," adding, "If he offends again, charges will be brought against him. Drunkards are not wanted in the Medical Department. Surgeon Barton is enjoined to report Asst. Surgeon Upshur whenever he is under the influence of liquor."[83] Concerning a different issue, Moore reminded Carrington of the court martial of certain surgeons: "The appointment of the wives of Medical Officers . . . should not be countenanced by Surgeons in charge of hospitals."[84]

The services of a contract physician could be terminated if his skills were no longer needed or if his superiors found him incompetent or dishonest. As a pool of available contract physicians developed, the Medical Department continued to contract only the most talented. In February 1863 Carrington directed Dr. McCaw to forward to him the names of eight acting assistant surgeons on duty at Chimborazo: "You will select the names of those who, in your judgment, are the least efficient."[85]

Promotions to a higher rank or office were based mainly upon merit. Samuel Stout provided a good example of this. Stout received his promotion from post surgeon to medical director of hospitals of the Army of Tennessee largely because of the quality of his hospital, seen by General Braxton Bragg during an impromptu inspection, and of this he later observed, "I well remember the chagrin manifested by many medical men and professors of colleges from the cities, who unmistakably manifested their disappointment. Some I heard of as saying 'Who in the hell is that fellow *Stout?*'"[86] Stout quickly proved himself, however, and gained the respect of his fellow surgeons. In many ways Stout's management style was similar to that of McCaw. Schroeder-Lein observed, "Stout . . . inspired cooperation from his subordinates by his own actions and attitudes. He set an example of obedience and subordination to his own superiors. He also set an example by his seeming tireless endeavors for 'professional self-improvement,' and his zeal for duty."[87]

A review of the evidence suggests that most Confederate physicians were competent doctors who received even further training while in the army. In fact, the standards set by the Confederate Medical Department and its medical boards caused many hospitals to face shortages in the number of doctors and other medical staff available. However, the standards did ensure the quality of those who worked in the field and hospitals of the Confederate medical service.

Little specific information is known about the physicians who served at Chimborazo. According to Phoebe Pember, they were a mixed group. On one hand she reported, "There were many sensible, kind-hearted efficient men among the surgeons who gave their time and talents generously to further the comfort and well-being of their patients."[88] On the other hand, however, she did not think as highly as some of the other physicians. Early in the war Pember wrote that not all the young surgeons were gentlemen and described how these doctors and the nurses in their wards would cover for each other when absent. When the doctors were "off on a frolic," the nurses would simply duplicate the diet lists and prescriptions of the day before; in appreciation, the doctors would give their nurses extra time off—unofficially, of course.[89] The situation seems to have improved later in the war. "A better educated class of surgeons was sent to fill fortunate vacancies," Pember noted.[90]

Chimborazo's records do reveal mentorship by the senior surgeons toward the ward surgeons. In one medical case book from Chimborazo No. 4, an assistant surgeon recorded daily reports on three patients admitted to his ward in February 1864. Surgeon W. A. Davis monitored his orders of these patients and advised the assistant surgeon to discontinue the use of a flaxseed poultice for one of them. Davis was evidently impressed by this physician; within a few weeks he transferred him to Ward F, a ward set aside exclusively for the more difficult wounded cases.[91]

Among the many doctors at Chimborazo there were, no doubt, many different personalities, strengths, and weaknesses. With such a large group working together daily, strengths could be shared and weaknesses minimized. Chimborazo's physicians served in an institution whose organization allowed mentorship and teamwork. Unlike doctors in field hospitals, Chimborazo's physicians had access to many second opinions in difficult cases, the latest medical knowledge, and specialists in Richmond. They had the luxury of a stationary hospital built on a medically sound architectural plan and one of the most effective systems of supply procurement of any Confederate hospital. They worked for an administrator who managed the facility according to what would improve patient care and who defined patient care in terms of the physical and mental well-being of the patient. And, if all else failed, they worked under the watchful eye of the hospital's matrons.

Although Chimborazo's physicians were definitely an indispensable group at the hospital, the hundreds of other workers were just as important. Matron Pember wrote, "Besides [the physicians], the hospital contained an endless horde of stewards and their clerks, surgeons' clerks; commissaries and their clerks; quartermasters and clerks; apothecaries and clerks; baggage-masters; forage-masters; cooks; bakers; carpenters; shoemakers; ward-inspectors; ambulance-drivers; and many more."[92] The matrons and nurses were also especially important because of their direct patient interaction. The next chapter will explore the roles of the managers of the wards, the nurses who performed the patient care, and the behind-the-scenes staff who kept Chimborazo running.

CHAPTER 3

The Staff

In the years before the Civil War, the staff of an army hospital consisted of a steward and a few detailed, convalescent patients. The steward performed the tasks of pharmacist, clerk, and general manager of the wards, and the detailed men provided all the nursing care and did the miscellaneous jobs such as cooking and cleaning. This system worked reasonably well in the small hospitals, which were really no more than clinics for soldiers who became ill. Even during the Mexican War, which brought some limited changes to hospitals, the staff remained basically the same.

The size and uniqueness of Chimborazo caused many changes to develop in the job descriptions of the hospital's staff. One steward could not possibly perform all the necessary duties required to care for a division hospital of six hundred patients. Problems arose with inadequate nursing care by detailed soldiers. Also, because Chimborazo was designated as an independent army post, the hospital needed numerous people to work in miscellaneous areas, such as the kitchens and blacksmith shop, where healthy soldiers were normally assigned on regular army posts. Obviously, a large number of strong, healthy workers was required to run and maintain operations at the hospital. However, the war's demand for the same type of men to serve on the front lines challenged McCaw's resourcefulness.

McCaw met the challenge by adapting old positions such as steward to fit the new situation. Tasks were broken down and assigned to as many men as were needed to perform them. New positions such as wardmaster and matron were created to perform new duties. To fill all these positions, McCaw hired free blacks, slaves, and women to supplement the detailed men he was allowed. Through his flexibility and open-mindedness, he staffed his hospital with workers who made his facility well known throughout the South.

Since Chimborazo Hospital did not open until the end of 1861, it was not the first Confederate hospital to employ blacks or women. It was, however, the first of the large division hospital complexes, and as such, its acquisition of workers provided a model of success that other large Confederate hospitals could follow.

Throughout the Civil War, approximately one thousand women served as nurses in Confederate hospitals; nine thousand served in Union hospitals. Those numbers do not include the large number of women who provided help temporarily when the battles occurred near their homes or who served unofficially for short periods of time.[1] The reason for the difference in the numbers between the North and the South is that the majority of persons who served as nurses in Confederate hospitals were male slaves, hired out by their masters. Most of the one thousand women mentioned above were white women who served as matrons in the South's hospitals.

The Confederate army initially copied the Union army's method for providing nursing care: enlisted men in the area of a hospital that needed nurses would be temporarily detailed to perform that duty. A common practice in field hospitals in the early months of the war was to detail a new set of men for nursing duty every few hours. A major problem with this practice, of course, was the men's lack of even basic skills in providing proper nursing care for their comrades. However, getting strong healthy men permanently assigned to the hospitals remained difficult because of the demand to have those men fighting on the front lines. Besides, very few nurses anywhere in the country had received any formal training in how to care for the sick or wounded. Nursing skill was seen mainly as a mixture of compassion, common sense, and hard work.

Initially, the situation was not much better in the Confederacy's general hospitals. Soldiers who were disabled or otherwise unable to be useful in battle were detailed to hospitals to serve as nurses. Many of these men were former patients who had partially recovered but had not yet gained enough strength to return to duty in the field; the common term for these men was "convalescent patients." Complaints about this system quickly arose from doctors and patients alike. Edmund Burke Haywood, surgeon-in-charge at a Raleigh hospital, expressed some of these sentiments to Surgeon General Moore: "It will be impossible to keep a hospital in fine order and the patients well cared for with broken down disabled men. . . . A disabled man cannot lift the sick, carry out the beds, scour the floor or sit up at night, or do many other things which are necessary in a well conducted hospital."[2]

Another problem arose when the detailed men recovered enough to return to duty. Surgeon R. L. Madison, who was in charge of the Orange Courthouse General Hospital, wrote to Dr. Thomas Williams, the medical director of Virginia, in October 1861, complaining about the frequent change of nurses in his hospital. Dr. Williams instructed Madison that he could request certain men to be formally detailed as nurses, entitling them to extra pay of twenty-five cents per day. However, even after Madison complied with regulations, he lost several of his detailed nurses a few months later when their field commanders decided they wanted them back.[3]

As the problems with using detailed enlisted men to serve as nurses soon became evident, the Confederate Congress approved an act on August 21, 1861, giving the secretary of war the power "To authorize the employment of Cooks and Nurses, other than enlisted men, or volunteers, for the Military Service." These new employees of Confederate hospitals were subject to military control and paid by the quartermasters a maximum of $18.50 per month, which was the same amount a soldier detailed on hospital duty would receive.[4] Some of these new positions were filled with white women, but most were filled by either free blacks or by slaves, hired out by their masters for one year at a time. When white women were hired, which was rare at this early point in the war, they were normally designated as "matrons," a position not alluded to in the congressional act and that paid only $6.00 per month.[5] Although conditions improved in hospitals with the new employees, a lack of training and a lack of supervision limited the level of improvement.

The varied duties of nurses required a strong stomach, a sturdy back, and a willingness to work hard. Usually, two or three nurses were assigned to each ward at Chimborazo. The head nurse's responsibilities included administering the medications ordered by the physicians, keeping track of his patients, and supervising the other nurses of his ward. The regulations of Winder Hospital also stated, "He will allow no patient to keep arms, accoutrements or knapsacks in his ward, nor to introduce any fruits or improper diet—and will be held responsible for the order, discipline, and cleanliness of his Ward."[6]

In addition to carrying out any medical treatments the physicians might order, the duties of nurses included bathing and feeding their patients and cleaning their wards. All patients at Chimborazo received full baths as soon as their condition permitted. Then, on a daily basis, nurses bathed patients' faces and necks, chests and arms, and legs and feet. At mealtimes, the nurses got the food for their bedridden patients from the matron's kitchen and then distributed it, feeding those who were unable to do so themselves. Nurses also cleaned the wards. Historian James H. Brewer explained, "The nurses were required to change the straw in the bed sacks at least once a month, and the beds had to be well beaten and thoroughly aired daily. Scouring the floor space occupied by the beds under one's care was also a responsibility of the nurse."[7]

McCaw preferred to assign white men as the head nurses of the wards at Chimborazo; the other two nurses were usually hired black workers. However, the ideal situation was rarely realized. In August of 1864, McCaw wrote to Medical Director Carrington requesting more nurses: "I have but 13 white nurses who are able to do effective service in the wards. . . . We require no less than one trusty man to each ward, and therefore require now 52 nurses."[8] To help alleviate the lack of white nurses, McCaw had apparently hired more black nurses. In July, after reporting the number of able-bodied black men employed at Chimborazo to Carrington, McCaw received a letter from Carrington informing him of the excess in the number of nurses at Chimborazo No. 1, No. 3, and No. 5.[9]

The January 29, 1862, report of the committee of a special congressional investigation noted many problems in the Medical Department. The committee was "deeply impressed with the inadequacy of the preparations and provisions for sick soldiers."[10] To remedy the situation, the committee suggested several changes, one of which was the establishment of a nursing corps. Their report stated, "Good nursing is of equal value to medical attention."[11] Actions on the committee's findings remained limited until later that year.

On September 27, 1862, the Confederate Congress passed "An act to better provide for the sick and wounded of the army in hospitals." This act allowed each hospital to employ two matrons, two assistant matrons, and as many nurses and cooks as might be needed, as well as a ward master for each ward. Because of an increasing awareness of and appreciation for women's talent for nursing, those in charge of hiring these newest additions to the hospitals were instructed to "[give] preference in all cases to females where their services may best serve the purpose."[12]

Many women had revealed their nursing talents in hospitals where they had worked as volunteers since the war began. Recognizing the demand for good nurses and remembering heroic stories of Florence Nightingale's work in Britain's Crimean War, women had volunteered their services as one way they could contribute to the war effort. Kate Cumming, a Southern volunteer who served as a nurse, stated, "I can not see what else we can do, as the war is certainly ours as well as that of the men. We can not fight, so must take care of those who do."[13] Other women worked as nurses in the hope of attending to a family member if he was wounded or became sick.

A hot debate—which occurred in both the North and the South and among both men and women—ensued concerning whether women should be allowed to nurse the soldiers. Many people thought that women were naturally too delicate to handle the horrors of wounds and disease, too sensitive to suffering, and too modest to dress the wounds or bathe the soldiers' bodies. Nursing male family members was one thing, but giving such personal care to complete strangers could not be allowed. Many women agreed with these objections and supported the war effort by rolling bandages, organizing charity bazaars, and contributing in other ways through their local aid societies.

Most of the women who served in Civil War hospitals agreed that under normal circumstances hospital work might be distasteful but that during the war they could not sit back and allow men to die because it might offend society's rules. In the closing pages of her memoirs, Phoebe Pember, who served at Chimborazo, expressed her opinion about "the distasteful [subject] that a woman must lose a certain amount of delicacy and reticence in filling any office in [a hospital]":

How can this be? There is no unpleasant exposure under proper arrangements, and if even there be, the circumstances which surround a wounded man, far from friends and home, suffering in a holy cause and dependent upon a woman for help, care, and sympathy, hallow and clear the atmosphere in which she labors. That woman must indeed be hard and gross, who lets one material thought lessen her efficiency. In the midst of suffering and death, hoping with those almost beyond hope in this world; praying by the bedside of the lonely and heart-stricken; closing the eyes of boys hardly old enough to realize man's sorrows, much less suffer by man's fierce hate, a woman *must* soar beyond the conventional modesty considered correct under different circumstances. If the ordeal does not chasten and purify her nature, if the contemplation of suffering and endurance does not make her wiser and better, and if the daily fire through which she passes does not draw from her nature the sweet fragrance of benevolence, charity, and love,— then indeed a hospital has been no fit place for her![14]

The initial way that women tended to the South's sick and wounded soldiers was to work collectively through various local charity groups to organize make-shift hospitals. As Moore began to consolidate many of these smaller facilities into larger general hospitals such as Chimborazo, many of the women who had volunteered their time and efforts to the smaller hospitals began to focus their attention on helping in other ways. As the lack of good nursing care in the general hospitals became more evident, the Medical Department realized how important some volunteer women had been as watchdog figures in the hospitals and how disruptive other volunteers could be without supervision. The need for permanent supervision of the hospitals' nurses and the visitors prompted the passage of the act of September 27, 1862.

Nursing care in Confederate hospitals did improve as a result of the act. Although few women sought positions as nurses because of societal pressures, some remained determined to serve their country by tending its sick and wounded heroes. The lack of a centralized office or agency in the South for women who wished to apply to be nurses hindered their efforts in obtaining a position. Women in the Union could apply to Dorothea Dix, who served as the superintendent of women nurses for the Union army, or to the United States Sanitary Commission to receive an appointment. In contrast, Confederate women wrote letters of application to area hospitals or to individuals they knew who were serving in the Medical Department. Many of the women who applied to work in the hospitals were hired as matrons, and as such they greatly contributed to the growing respectability of life in the hospitals.

Recognizing the reticence that Southern women might have with regard to paid nursing duties, the act of September 27 provided "for the permanent detail of soldiers as nurses and ward masters in case a sufficient number of these attendants could not be obtained outside the military service."[15] With this authority in hand, surgeons began choosing their detailed men more carefully, hoping to train these men and retain their services for the duration of the war. Yet, because of the increasing demand for able-bodied men in the field, the Surgeon General's Office agreed that such men should be on the front lines, leaving only the disabled to work in the hospitals. Chimborazo received instruction to "return any men not disabled to duty in the field" on June 5, 1863.[16] At this point, the hospital had 163 detailed men serving there, although it is not known how many of these men were considered able-bodied or how many disabled.[17]

Black Employees

Because of the difficulty in obtaining healthy soldiers to serve as nurses, Chimborazo and Confederate hospitals throughout the South relied heavily on black employees to fill its ranks. Blacks made up over a third of Richmond's prewar population. Of Richmond's 38,000 inhabitants in 1859, there were 11,699 slaves and 2,576 free blacks.[18] Many blacks had been hired out by their masters to the city's numerous factories and other businesses. Ernest Furgurson described Richmond in 1859 as "the most important industrial complex in the South," citing its bustling trade of such commodities as tobacco and wheat and naming such businesses as the Tredegar Iron Works, the Crenshaw Woolen Mills, the Franklin Paper Mill, seven major flour mills, and fifty tobacco factories.[19] Blacks provided much of the labor for those businesses. Many workers were under yearly contracts, negotiated on New Year's Day, while others were owned outright by businesses. More than twenty major slave auction companies prospered in Richmond. According to Furgurson, "By 1859–60, sales in Richmond were running at more than $4 million a year." This made the slave trade the city's biggest business by dollar volume.[20] The city had an extensive black code, but those repressive laws still allowed more independence for its blacks when compared to slaves who lived on plantations. "[T]he city's domestic servants and artisans," wrote Furgurson, "were urban sophisticates, often fashionably dressed on Sundays, en route to a church of their own. Slave and free blacksmiths, barbers, cooks, draymen, and tobacco-factory hands were hired out by the thousands, earning wages and socializing among themselves, almost as if they were not black at all."[21]

When the war erupted and Richmond's economy adjusted to the Confederate war effort, most of the city's slaves and free blacks changed jobs. Tobacco factories and other businesses closed, and war factories and the armory began hiring more workers so that they could run multiple shifts. Tredegar Iron Works immediately shifted to a seven-day work week. Richmond's expanding population needed cooks and maids in their homes and workers for the new service-oriented businesses in the city. Also, hospitals needed black workers to serve as nurses, cooks, and other laborers; many found the blacks who worked in these positions indispensable.[22]

From its beginning, Chimborazo's reliance upon slave labor was evident. Slave labor under the supervision of McCaw and the quartermaster's department built the facility and afterwards provided most of the labor to run the hospitals. On May 17, 1862, McCaw informed Moore of his desperate need to retain the slaves working at Chimborazo:

> I have at this time only two hundred and fifty-six cooks & nurses in my Hospitals, to take care of nearly four thousand sick soldiers and the owners of these slaves are threatening to remove them to the interior of the country to avoid losing them. I am confident a large number will be removed in a few days unless measures are taken to prevent it. I therefore respectfully ask that these servants, with as many others as may be needed be immediately impressed, as it will be entirely impossible to continue the hospital without them.
>
> p.s. This subject requires immediate action.[23]

Moore responded the same day, telling McCaw that he had referred the matter to General Winder and stating, "If these negroes are permitted to leave, the hospitals will be abandoned & the sick left destitute of nurses."[24] The slaves were not allowed to leave.

This was not the first time that blacks had been impressed. As early as July 1861, the Richmond City Council authorized Mayor Joseph Carrington Mayo to impress free blacks to help construct the city's fortifications. The workers were paid eleven dollars per month, the same as army privates, and provided with food and drink. Recognizing the high demand for slave labor, the Confederate Congress passed legislation in February, 1862, allowing the impressment of free black men between eighteen and fifty years of age for up to six months. A similar law, passed in October 1862, allowed military commanders to impress slaves for up to two months. "The Confederate government would pay their owners $16 a month per slave and provision the laborers as if they were soldiers. Owners would also be compensated for slaves who died or were hurt while serving, or ran away to the enemy."[25]

Most of Chimborazo's black employees were slave men, although the hospital's records do show that women and free blacks worked there as well. By the summer of 1863, Chimborazo No. 1 employed 120 blacks; only 12 were free. Most of the hospital's black workers served in the wards, nursing and cleaning. Many other black employees worked in the laundry or the kitchens, where apparently a few women served as the chief cook in their division's kitchen. Blacks also served at the soaphouses, the bakery, the icehouse, the dairy, and the farm; on Chimborazo's canal boat; and in any other position where manual labor was needed.[26]

The wages of the black workers depended on their skills. At the beginning of the war, Chimborazo paid as little as $60.00 per year for young men who served as assistants to the nurses and cooks. Laundresses' monthly pay rose from $8.00 in 1861 to $12.00 in late 1862 and $18.50 in 1863. By 1863, cooks and nurses were paid $25.00 per month. The Confederate Congress had decided that the pay of cooks and nurses (who were not enlisted men or volunteers) could not exceed that of soldiers detailed to hospital duty. In November 1861, a soldier's salary was $11.00 per month, plus $.25 per day extra for hospital duty, totaling $18.50 per month. All hospital attendants, military and civilian, slave and free, were paid by the quartermaster's department.[27]

By the end of the war, of course, these amounts had escalated. At the top of Chimborazo's pay scale for black workers was a free black man named George Cox, who worked as a nurse, and a free black woman named Candis, who worked as a cook. They each received $240 for their services to Chimborazo No. 2 in 1862. Cox and Candis were paid $400 in 1864. In addition to providing statistics about wages, Chimborazo's records also reveal the long tenure of some black employees at the facility. Although the existing records are sketchy, some blacks apparently served at the hospital from the time it opened until it closed in 1865.[28] In most wage agreements the hospital provided the food and clothing. However, especially toward the end of the war, other arrangements were sometimes worked out. In January 1864 McCaw wrote to a Mrs. Harwood, "I will take your servant Robert at four hundred dollars and rations, but you [are] to furnish the clothing."[29]

Some of the black employees were owned by Chimborazo's medical officers. Surgeon-in-Chief McCaw owned at least two: Hannibal, employed at Chimborazo No. 3, and Bob, employed at Chimborazo No. 2. Dr. G. E. Alsop owned nine slaves, Dr. E. H. Smith owned six, and Dr. P. F. Browne owned three. According to James H. Brewer in his work *Confederate Negro*, "If the number of slave nurses owned by physicians is evidence that they held some nursing training, then Chimborazo was indeed fortunate. In 1863 the hospital's muster rolls listed 15 medical doctors eligible to receive $7,000 for the services of 35 slave nurses."[30]

The sources of Chimborazo's other black employees varied. In late 1862, Brewer stated, "newspapers throughout [Virginia] advertised that Chimborazo seeks 'to hire, for the year, 250 men, women, and boys (over 12 years of age), as cooks and nurses.'"[31] Many individuals responded to the ads, writing to McCaw of their desire to hire out a few of their slaves. C. W. M. Hubball wrote, "[H]aveing [sic] seen your advertisement this morning for Sevts in your hospital would say I have 3 — one a first rate cook & two boys, 18 years of age if you have no cases of smallpox & will return them if such should be the case."[32] Quite a few "agents" helped supply the hospital with slaves. "The muster rolls of the hospital disclosed the names of many agents in the Richmond area," Brewer wrote, "including Clopton and Lyne, P. M. Tabb and Son, Turpin and Yarbrough, and E. D. Eacho. One agent, James H. Grant, supplied over 50 slave nurses and cooks."[33]

Evidently, the slaves and other black employees were treated well at Chimborazo. As Brewer noted, "Dr. McCaw was extremely perceptive as to the Negroes' needs for well-being and happiness."[34] McCaw recognized the importance of good employees to his facility and worked diligently throughout the war to provide for them the best he could. One way he did this was by interceding on their behalf to exempt them from outside obligations. At the beginning of 1863, he wrote to Colonel J. F. Gilmen, chief of the Engineering Bureau, explaining the necessity of exempting the free blacks at Chimborazo from working on the fortifications being built around Richmond. Colonel Gilmen and his superior, Colonel W. A. Stevens, chief of the Construction Division of North Virginia, did not agree with McCaw on the matter. McCaw appealed to Medical Director William Carrington, who not only supported McCaw, but ordered all surgeons-in-charge to obtain exemptions for the free blacks working in their hospitals as well.[35]

One way McCaw showed his appreciation to his black workers was by giving them extra pay for working during the holidays.[36] By 1864 Moore had evidently decided that McCaw's idea was a good one. That year he authorized the surgeons-in-charge at all military hospitals "to pay their hired slaves one dollar per diem during Christmas week, using the Hospital fund for the purpose."[37]

Matrons

The matrons became important managers and supervisors at the hospitals. The matron's duties focused on keeping the hospital clean and orderly and preparing the food for the patients. According to the act passed in September 1862, the matrons were "to exercise a superintendence over the entire domestic economy of the hospital, to take charge of such delicacies as may be provided for the sick, to apportion them out as required, to see that the food or diet is properly prepared," and to carry out "all such other duties as may be necessary."[38] The matrons, according to Pember, "had no official recognition, ranking even below stewards from a military point of view."[39]

The major qualifications for matrons were a pleasant demeanor, ladylike behavior, intelligence, and a willingness to work hard. Matrons were usually widows who had no dependent children and who needed respectable employment. Nursing skills or experience were not necessarily required. Personal letters of recommendations were instrumental for a woman to gain a position as a matron. For example, William Alex Thorn wrote to McCaw about a Mrs. Ann T. Goodwin of Fredericksburg, a "widow of a former cashier of one the banks there—a refugee from home without means of support." Thorn wrote, "Mrs. Goodwin is a Lady of fine social position, intelligence, an old & excellent housekeeper & rather remarkable in Fredericksburg as a good nurse." At the end of the letter, Thorn added, "I would take it as a personal favor if you could give her the situation she seeks."[40]

Initially, many of the surgeons and stewards in the hospitals viewed the matrons warily; they did not think respectable women could handle the horrors of hospital life or contribute positively to hospital operations on a daily basis. When Phoebe Pember arrived at Chimborazo and reported to the main offices of the hospital, she overheard one of the men there say that "one of them had come."[41]

The number and distribution of matrons varied from one hospital to another. One head matron was assigned to each of Chimborazo's five divisions: Mrs. Eliza Bayler in No. 1, Mrs. Phoebe Pember in No. 2, Mrs. Elizabeth Brown in No. 3, Mrs. Mary R. Cassels in No. 4, and Mrs. Tschndi in No. 5. The head matrons received forty dollars per month, with board and lodging provided. Each division also had one or two assistant matrons, who received thirty-five dollars per month, and two or three ward matrons, who were paid thirty dollars per month.[42]

Chimborazo had one chief matron, Mrs. Doctor Minge, "serving the hospital at large."[43] Very little is known about Minge or her duties. It is possible that she served as the chief matron in charge of the general laundry. Her name was not listed in the register that listed all the other matrons, their assignments, and their dates of employment.

By comparison, Winder Hospital had one chief matron in charge of the laundry who oversaw six assistant matrons, two laundry men, and all the laundresses. Winder also had one chief matron for the "ladies' kitchen" of each division, who also supervised the three ward matrons allowed each of hospital's divisions.[44] In another smaller hospital, the chief matron of the laundry department had the help of only one assistant matron and the added responsibility of the care of the bath house.[45]

Phoebe Yates Pember, the head matron of Chimborazo No. 2, is one of the best-known women to have served as a matron in a Confederate hospital because she kept notes and a diary while at Chimborazo. She later compiled those notes into her memoirs, which were published. Her records provide a great deal of insight into life at Chimborazo, both at center stage and behind the scenes. Pember was born in 1823 into a "prosperous and cultured Jewish family of Charleston, South Carolina." Her father, Jacob Levy, was "a gentleman of leisure" and her mother, Fanny Yates, was originally from England. Phoebe Yates married Thomas Pember of Boston, who had spent much time in the South because of poor health. After her husband died from tuberculosis in 1861, she went to Savannah, where her parents had moved several years before. Not wanting to be dependent on her family, she accepted an offer brought to her in November 1862 by Mrs. George W. Randolph, the wife of the Confederate secretary of war, to serve as a matron in a Confederate hospital, although she acknowledged that it was "rather a startling proposition to a woman used to all the comforts of luxurious life."[46] Given the choice of serving at Cotoosa Springs Hospital in Georgia or Chimborazo Hospital, she chose "the Richmond one, because it was divided among half a dozen ladies who would be companionable perhaps."[47]

After reporting for duty and being shown to her rooms she began trying to prepare the first meal for the six hundred patients on the matron's diet list. To do this task, she recalled, "A stove was unearthed; very small, very rusty, and fit only for a family of six."[48] She soon discovered that "[t]his state of affairs was only the result of accident and some misunderstanding. The surgeon of my hospital naturally thought I had informed myself of the power vested in my [sic] by virtue of my position, and having some experience, would use the rights given me by the law passed by Congress, to arrange my own department; and I, on reading that bill, could only understand that the office was one that dovetailed the duties of housekeeper and cook, nothing more."[49] She quickly learned how to requisition needed items for her kitchen but did not understand the full measure of her potential authority for several more days:

> [M]y office did not rise above that of chief cook, for I dared not leave my kitchen unattended for a moment, till Doctor James B. McCaw, one day, passing the window, and seeing me seated on a low bench peeling potatoes, appeared much surprised, and inquired where my cooks were. Explanations followed, a copy of hospital rules was sent for, and authority found to provide the matron's department with suitable attendants.[50]

The attendants for the matron's department, most of whom she hired, included the assistant matrons, the cooks, and the laundresses.

The major task of the head matron was to cook the foods for the invalids in her division. (The patients who could walk were required to eat in the "big kitchen" where the steward's cooks provided the food.) She would receive the orders for the patients after the surgeons made their morning rounds, when they could make changes to the patients' diets. Afterwards, "[t]he chief matron sat at her table, the diet lists arranged before her. . . . Any necessary instructions of the surgeons were noted and attended to, sometimes accompanied with observations of her own. . . . The orders ran somewhat in this fashion: 'Chicken soup for twenty—beef tea for forty—tea and toast for fifty.'"[51] She then sent for the necessary ingredients from the storerooms, or for substitutions if certain items were not available, so the cooking could begin.

One adjustment in cooking for so many men was changing recipies to meet the common tastes of the group. Many men were reluctant to eat something that looked, smelled, or tasted unfamiliar to them. Pember encountered this difficulty with the very first meal she made for her patients—chicken soup, which she was convinced needed the "sick man's parsley" to be complete. After handing a bowl of the soup to her first patient, she waited for his reaction: "A long painful gulp, a 'judematical' shake of the head, *not* in the affirmative, and the bowl traveled slowly back to my extended hand. 'My mammy's soup was not like that,' he whined. 'But I might worry a little down if it war'n't for them *weeds* a-floating round.'"[52]

Another problem was special requests. As Pember recalled, "If an invalid craved any particular dish the nurse mentioned the want, and if not contrary to the surgeon's order, it, or its nearest approximation was allowed him."[53] The first step in filling the request was to discover what exactly the patient wanted. Items like buttermilk, which was commonly craved by wounded patients, was easy enough to figure out, but it took a while for Pember to discover what constituted "sweet soup" or "sour soup." A detailed description of the dish's contents or sometimes even a recipe in a letter from the patient's home might be needed to fill the request. Once a dish had been determined, "the greatest difficulty in granting these desires was that tastes became contagious, and whatever one patient asked for, his neighbor and the one next to him, and so on throughout the wards, craved also, and it was impossible to decide upon whom to draw a check."[54]

Still another problem was finding something nutritious that the patient would eat and that also met the doctor's approval. A nurse reported to Pember that a patient named Jones refused to eat the tea and toast ordered for him. "[The doctor] . . . said Jones was out of his head, and Jones says the doctor is a fool."[55] The matron, at this point, usually approached both parties to try to work out some compromise that would fulfill the doctor's orders as well as provide some nourishment to the patient.

However challenging the task of cooking for a diverse group of sick and wounded men was, the role of the matron expanded a great deal during the course of the war. One of the most troublesome duties for Confederate matrons was the supervision of the hospital's liquor supply. The demand for liquor, for use as medication and recreation, was high at the onset of the war and only increased during the duration of the conflict. Since the use and abuse of liquor was so common during the first year of the war, the Confederate Congress sought to regulate its distribution in hospitals with the 1862 hospital bill. That act categorized liquors with other "luxuries" and placed those items under the control of the matron's department in hospitals. The matron was to allocate the necessary amounts of liquor that the patients needed after receiving a physician's order for the valued substance.[56]

Although the orders were in place, the battle for control of the monthly whiskey barrel was only decided as the matrons of hospitals asserted their authority as provided for by Congress. Matron Pember described this struggle as "a long and bitterly waged contest . . . which eventually became a symbol of authority in a tussle between the male and female contingents of the hospital staff."[57] As Pember gained more confidence in her abilities and the authority of her position, she took a stand on her right to control the whiskey barrel. The following is her account of the battle that ensued:

> [T]he monthly barrel of whiskey which I was entitled to draw still remained at the dispensary under the guardianship of the apothecary and his clerks, and quarts and pints were issued through any order coming from surgeons or their substitutes, so that the contents were apt to be gone long before I was entitled to draw more, and my sick would suffer for want of the stimulant. There were many suspicious circumstances connected with this *institution;* for the monthly barrel was an institution and a very important one.
>
>   . . . I referred to the hospital bill passed by Congress . . . and in an evil moment, such as tempted Pandora to open the fatal casket assailed me, and despatched [*sic*] the bill, flanked by a formal requisition for the liquor. An answer came in the shape of the head surgeon. He declared I would find 'the charge most onerous,' that 'whiskey was required at all hours, sometimes in the middle of the night, and even if I remained at the hospital, he would not like me disturbed,' 'it was constantly needed for medicinal purposes,' 'he was responsible for its proper application;' but I was not convinced, and withstood all argument and persuasion. He was proverbially sober himself, but I was aware why both commissioned and non-commissioned officers opposed violently the removal of the liquor to my quarters. So, the printed law being at hand for reference, I nailed my colors to the mast, and that evening all the liquor was in my pantry and the key in my pocket.[58]

The controversy over this action prompted Pember to appeal to McCaw for a final ruling on the matter. He settled the question at Chimborazo hospitals once and for all when he ruled that "the liquor was intended exclusively for the use of patients, and should be used through a prescription accompanied by a written order . . . and that [the head matron] was personally responsible for the quantity confided to [her] care, and must each month produce the surgeon's receipts to balance with the number of gallons drawn from the medical purveyor."[59]

Even though the question was officially resolved, the matrons continued to face small challenges over the distribution of whiskey throughout the war. Pember remembered some of the more annoying methods used in her memoirs. One was "sending a negro boy with a cup and a simple request for whiskey, as if it was the most natural act in the world." After politely refusing to grant the request without a written physician's order, she would send the boy away, only to have him return in the same manner, still without an order. This occurred "half a dozen times consecutively"—usually until she lost her temper and sent back a "brief but sharp note."[60] Another routine challenge occurred as follows:

> A quart bottle of whiskey would be ordered by the officer of the day
> for each ward, for night use, so that it would be ready at hand should
> any of the patients need this stimulant during the night. The next
> morning, on inquiring being made, there had been no cases requiring
> its use, but the bottles would be empty, and expostulation on my part
> be met with explanations that the rats (who were a very plague), had
> knocked the bottles over. . . . [T]he surgeon in charge would be
> appealed to, hear all sides, and favor none.[61]

The task of hiring and supervising the assistant matrons and ward matrons also fell to the head matron of a division. Although most matrons who came to Chimborazo remained there throughout most of the war, finding pleasant, reliable women to serve as matrons could be a problem—one that Pember experienced on several occasions. "[M]y choice," she recalled, "hesitated between ladies of education and position, who I knew would be willing to aid me, and the common class of respectable servants. The latter suited best, because it was to be supposed they would be more amenable to authority."[62] The first woman she had problems with evidently did not understand the nature of the position. Pember stated, "She had hardly left my kitchen when she returned with all the drinks, and a very indignant face. . . . She asserted loudly that she was a decent woman, and 'was not going anywhere in a place where a man sat up on his bed in his shirt.'"[63]

The second problematic employee, "a plausible, light-haired, light-eyed, and light complexioned Englishwoman" named Mrs. Stickney, was more difficult.[64] Unsatisfied with the quarters provided her, this petite woman partitioned off an eight-foot-by-ten-foot section of Ward E, moved her seven trunks in, and declared the area to be her quarters. When Pember tried to explain that this was unacceptable because of medical concerns about ventilation and for obvious reasons of respectability, the woman refused to leave. Pember appealed to Dr. Habersham for help, but he refused, saying that the woman was under her supervision. At Pember's request, the steward and a strong assistant began "to eject the new tenant. . . . [Then Mrs. Stickney] arose and rolled up her sleeves, advancing upon him as he receeded down the ward. The sick and wounded men roared with laughter, cheering her on, and she remained mistress of the field."[65] That evening at dinner, "whenever [the problematic matron] came across a bone in hash or stew, or indeed anything that displeased her, she took it in her fingers and dashed it upon the floor. . . . The surgeons stood laughing, in groups, the men crowded to the windows because of the belligerant power, and a *coup-d'etat* became necessary."[66] First, Pember sent for the carpenter and had him tear down the matron's room; then, the woman, reportedly drunk by this time, was put in Pember's ambulance and sent away. The next day the woman appealed to Medical Director Carrington and returned to Chimborazo by noon, with an order to "retain [her] in your Hospl, until she is able to secure a situation."[67] Surgeon S. E. Habersham explained to McCaw that the woman had been discharged, "finding her insubordinate and a pest and complained of on all sides. . . . [S]he is a dangerous character about a hospital."[68] McCaw had to explain the situation to Carrington so that the woman could be sent away permanently.[69]

Other, smaller challenges faced matrons on a daily basis. Over time, matrons developed a protective shell to keep their ladylike sensibilities intact as they experienced strange and unpleasant situations. In 1863 Pember concluded a letter to her sister by writing, "I must say goodbye as the Doctor has just come to lance a great abcess I have on my arm that has almost crazed me. You don't know how courageous the constant sight of amputations make one—you look upon anything less as trifling."[70] The next year Pember wrote of three mentally disturbed men who had been assigned to her division—"one of whom has a chronic affection for pulling off all his clothes the moment I go into his Ward."[71]

Although matrons were discouraged from providing nursing care for the patients, they stepped beyond their normal bounds in times of crisis. Pember's first experience in this realm occurred one night after the surgeons had left and the wounded from a nearby battle started arriving at Chimborazo. "[G]iving Miss G. orders to make an unlimited supply of coffee, tea, and stimulants, armed with lint, bandages, castile soap, and a basin of warm water, I made my first essays in the surgical line. I had been spectator often enough to be skillful. . . . From bed to bed till long past midnight, the work continued. Fractured limbs were bathed, washed free from blood and left for surgeons to set."[72] Pember and other matrons tried to limit the medical care they offered, because of the contempt with which many surgeons treated their efforts or suggestions. However, she also noted:

But antagonism was not always the rule. There were many sensible, kind-hearted efficient men among the surgeons who gave their time and talents generously to further the comfort and well-being of their patients,—men who would let me work hand in hand with them, the nurse with the doctor, and listen kindly and respectfully to my suggestions, if they were not calculated to benefit science.[73]

Some matrons did develop and exert their authority more than others. One of Winder Hospital's matrons changed a patient's diet orders at his request in order to help him regain his strength. That action could have been seen by some surgeons as a threat.[74]

Even more important than the direct medical care the matrons provided was their watchfulness over any questionable care that their patients might receive. In one situation a man with a crushed ankle had been transferred to Chimborazo after having it treated. That night a nurse reported to Pember that the patient "had a burning fever, and complained of the fellow leg instead of the injured one." Pember remembered, "I determined to look at him in spite of orders [to leave him undisturbed], his sufferings appearing so great, and finding the foot and leg above and below the splint perfectly well, the thought of examining the fellow leg suggested itself. It was a most shocking sight—swollen, inflamed and purple—the drunken surgeon had set the wrong leg!"[75] Immediate action was taken to soothe the proper ankle and the patient remained very much attached to the matron, and wary of surgeons, while at the hospital. "No surgeon in the hospital could persuade him to swallow anything in the shape of food unless I sanctioned the order, and a few kindly words, or an encouraging nod would satisfy and please him."[76]

A female presence in the wards, in the shape of a caring matron, made the men feel more at ease in their unfamiliar surroundings. Matrons presented a motherly figure to whom the men could relate. Pember described herself as "always dressed in Georgia homespun, often the worse for wear, leather shoes, worsted gloves, and half the time with a skillet or coffee-pot in my hands."[77] The matrons' concern for the patients was a feature of good medical care that was only beginning to be understood. McCaw stressed the importance of good morale among the patients at the hospital, but achieving the goal of providing personal attention to the patients was largely left to the matron. Many on the hospital's staff quickly learned to look to the matrons when a feminine touch could help ease a patient. Pember reported, "Feminine sympathy being much more demonstrative than masculine . . . the nurses often summoned me when only the surgeon was needed."[78]

Through their influence and their kindness, the matrons could also calm the patients in times of crisis. Miss Emily Mason, a matron at Winder Hospital, remembered an incident when two hundred men, hungry for bread, tore down the hospital's bakery. She controlled the crisis by reminding the men of her kindness to them, including her willingness to stew some rats when the cook refused to prepare such a dish.[79] Mason's words comforted the men, because they realized that she was on their side and would give them as much food as was available.

Most matrons received very little direct praise for their work. Pember remembered that the few compliments she received "were noticeable from their originality and novelty."[80] One of the more memorable of these came from a "rough looking Texan," who told her that she was "as pretty as a pair of red shoes with green strings."[81] The connection she made with her patients provided some reward in itself. In a letter to her sister Eugenia, Pember wrote, "I bring comfort, strength and I believe happiness to many sick beds daily and lie down at night with a happy consciousness of time well and unselfishly spent."[82] Her patients' actions also contributed to a self-recognition of her worth:

> The early and comforting visit to the sick after their feverish, restless
> night; when even if there was no good to be effected, they would
> feel the kindness, and every man's head would be thrust out of the
> bed-clothes as by one impulse, and jealously evinced when a longer
> pause by one bedside than another would arouse the feeling. Often
> has the ward-master recalled me when at the distance of a quarter of
> a mile from his ward, at the request of a patient, and when going back
> to find out what was wanted, a hearty convalescent would explain
> that I had passed through and omitted to speak to him.[83]

Pember experienced another example of the connection between herself and her patients after a confrontation with a critical patient, a man "who ate too many luxury pickles." She wrote, "[T]hat afternoon came a formal apology, written in quite an elegant style, and signed by every man in the ward, except the pickle man."[84] When a large group of patients left her wards at the same time, she missed them and "felt a great repugnance to visiting [the new patients]" until she became familiar with them and they understood who she was.[85] The connection she made with a few patients prompted them to write to her after they had left Chimborazo; one group of soldiers from Maryland, for whom Pember felt a special concern, was especially thoughtful in this regard.[86]

Pember's own awareness of the connection between herself and her patients was heightened when health problems forced her to obtain a month-long leave of absence from Chimborazo in 1864. She wrote, "It had been like tearing body and soul apart, when necessity compelled me to leave the hospital, from which I had never been separated but one day in nearly four years. . . . A visit to the wards did not tend to strengthen my wavering resolves. The first invalid to whom I communicated the news of my intended departure burst into a passion of tears."[87]

Through their hard work and caring attention to the needs of the patients, many matrons proved themselves to the medical officers. However, certain prejudices against the matrons did linger. Moore provided an example of this in a letter to McCaw:

> It has been reported to this Bureau that one of the Matrons of your hospital is accustomed to entertain company at dinner.
>
> You will make enquiry as to whether this is habitual with any of your Chief Matrons. It is so easy for them to become wasteful and extravagant, that the utmost vigilence is necessary to ascertain whether the governmental supplies are not misapplied.[88]

In the larger scheme of things, however, very few individuals who had seen the work and effect of the matrons could dispute their value to the success of the hospitals.

Stewards

Besides the surgeon-in-charge and the matron, the other indispensable manager in a well-run hospital was the steward. The hands-on manager of each of Chimborazo's five divisions was the chief steward (also called the mess steward), who held the rank of sergeant. The evolution of the position of steward provides another interesting example of how the medical staffs of hospitals changed because of the Civil War. Before the war the steward was generally the pharmacist. Since mixing the drugs was not a full-time task, this individual also handled nursing and other miscellaneous duties in the hospitals. It was not until 1856 that men serving as stewards were permanently attached to the U.S. Army medical department.[89]

Early in the nineteenth century, the position of apothecary in hospitals was filled by medical apprentices, who used the position to gain hands-on experience in compounding medications as well as in going on rounds and treating patients. As apothecaries gained more responsibilities, hospitals and dispensaries began to choose full-time pharmaceutical practitioners to fill these positions and required them to stay in their workrooms instead of going on rounds. Besides their pharmaceutical duties, apothecaries became important managers in hospitals. Because of the weight of their responsibilities, many hospitals began to require character references before hiring an apothecary. In 1819 the bylaws of New York Hospital "required not only testimonials on an applicant's behalf, but also a $250 bond to ensure 'faithful performance of the duties of his office, and that he will not cease to perform the duties of this office, without giving two months notice of his intention to leave his employment.'"[90]

In the late 1830s and early 1840s, the apothecary's status began to deteriorate just as that of the regular physician did. Their customers' increasing requests for patent medicines prompted many apothecaries to expand their assortment of these items, which hurt relations between pharmacists and physicians. Physicians also resented the fact that pharmacists were more commonly granting customers' requests for refills on certain items without their doctor's approval and were giving more medical advice from the counters of their shops.[91]

The position of steward changed with the coming of the war and the establishment of large hospitals. On May 16, 1861, the Confederate Congress authorized the position of hospital steward, with the rank of sergeant. Initially, stewards were to serve as druggists, managers of the wards, and custodians of hospital property.[92] As the various responsibilities became too great for one person to handle, a distinction arose in the general hospitals between an apothecary, a mess steward, and the main clerk of a division, although men doing any of the above tasks were officially referred to as stewards. Each division or hospital normally had at least one man in each position.

Chimborazo's records sometimes list more than three stewards, but many of those additional men were probably students who attended the Medical College of Virginia and sought to gain practical experience about medical treatment and hospital life by working and living at Chimborazo. Several letters in Chimborazo's records were requests to McCaw to find steward positions for young men wanting to attend lectures at the Medical College of Virginia.[93] Existing records indicate that allowances were made at Chimborazo for larger steward numbers in order to accommodate these medical students. In late 1864, when troop strengths were dangerously low, Carrington ordered McCaw to "report the names of any Hospital Steward, not Students of Medicine, not required at the Hospl [sic] under your charge."[94]

The mess steward worked directly under the surgeon-in-charge of the hospital. As a sergeant he had to take orders from the assistant surgeons, but he could appeal to the surgeon-in-charge if he thought the orders were extreme. In a letter to Carrington, McCaw explained the position of the mess stewards at Chimborazo. "My five leading Stewards or managers were selected by their knowledge of good meat & good cooking & not because they were learned in pharmacy. Their duty is to manage negros [sic] and cook provisions."[95] An expanded description of the duties of the mess steward occurs in the regulations of Winder Hospital:

> It shall be the duty of the Mess Steward to take due care of the Hospital
> Stores and Supplies; to prepare the provision returns; to receive and
> distribute rations; to control the convalescent kitchen and dining
> room; to furnish to the pantry of the ladies' kitchen upon the requisi-
> tion of the Chief Matron, such delicacies . . . which can be purchased

with the Hospital fund; to keep a record of the transactions of his department, and to render a written report of same to the Commssary [*sic*] of the Hospital and to his Division Surgeon at the end of every month.[96]

The stewards also supervised the wardmasters and nurses of the hospital. Phoebe Pember provided another view of the steward's duties: "The steward of a hospital cannot define exactly what his duties are, the difficulty being to find out what they are not. Whenever it has to be decided who has to fill a disagreeable office, the choice invariably falls upon the steward."[97] Before the act of September 1862, the steward's responsibilities had also included the tasks given to the head matron.

Stewards were considered key managers of hospitals. When Carrington wanted to open a receiving hospital in May 1864, he asked McCaw for any attendants Chimborazo could spare to fill the number of required personnel to do so: "3 Hosp Stewards, 45 Ward Masters & nurses, 12 Cooks." Carrington added that he "would like very much to get one of your Stewards, who is accustomed to managing your laundry arrangements with outsiders."[98] The importance of stewards to hospitals was further revealed in a July 8, 1864, circular from the Surgeon General's Office. It stated that "stewards were the only able-bodied white men between the ages of seventeen and forty-five employed in hospitals who were exempted from field duty."[99]

As the Medical Department became aware of the general distrust that had begun to develop about mess stewards, the surgeon general decided to order the examination of all hospital stewards. Carrington appointed a board of three surgeons that began to convene daily from 11:00 A.M. to 2:00 P.M. at General Hospital No. 10 in Richmond to conduct the examinations. Carrington then summoned the stewards on duty in Virginia, several at a time, to Richmond for their examinations.[100] The board was instructed to furnish a written report of the results of each exam as soon as possible after conducting it. The general information on the report included the person's full name, date of appointment as steward, whether enlisted or civilian, where he was serving on duty and where he had principally served, and "his *physical* competency for duty in field or Hospital." Through the examination process, the board investigated "*the moral fitness* of the Steward for his office. 'He should be temperate, honest, and every way reliable and *known to be such*.'" These qualifications were to be determined through the presentation of written testimonials from the officers he had served under, as well as any adverse reports received about the steward. If any question remained about the steward's moral fitness, the board was admonished to delay its final report until it could communicate with his past and present supervisors.[101]

The last phase of the examination was to determine the knowledge and skills of the men and whether they could properly fulfill the duties of steward. McCaw wrote to Carrington concerning the skills section, stating, "It should be remembered in this examination of stewards about to take place that I have here two classes of them both called hospital stewards (for want of any other name) who are engaged in very different occupations. . . . To examine [the mess stewards] on Pharmacy will be to lose me their services which can not be replaced."[102] Carrington decided to have the board of examiners distinguish among the positions of steward—mess steward, apothecary, or clerk—in which an applicant could serve.

The examinations quickly revealed the various talents and deficiencies of the stewards. The board found some men capable of serving in any steward position, and it rejected other men entirely. Most applicants were determined to be qualified in the area in which they were currently serving. Of William H. Smith, a civilian steward hired in 1862 to work at Chimborazo No. 3, the board reported, "Examination satisfactory as Mess Steward. No knowledge of Pharmacy." William P. Brewer's report read "incapable of field service. . . . Acting as apothecary, has not discharged any other duties of H. Steward. Examination Satisfactory for Apothecary only." Some men were probably surprised by the board's findings. James Johnson, an apothecary serving at Winder Hospital, was a druggist by occupation but rejected by the board as "not sufficiently intelligent nor skilled in pharmacy." George W. Muse, an apothecary at Howard's Grove Hospital who had worked as a physician before the war, was rejected as an apothecary and approved only for the position of mess steward. In a few reports the board praised those who particularly impressed them. Of Burke Archer, the twenty-five-year-old apothecary for the officers in private quarters, the board wrote, "We found him the best informed apothecary that has appeared before this board up to this time." These examinations helped to remove incompetent stewards from their positions and limit their future assignments to duties they could properly perform.[103]

The distinctions regarding the different kinds of stewards remained in place after the war in large hospitals. The separation between the mess steward and the apothecary steward would later assist pharmacists as they began efforts to develop their skills into a profession. Near the end of the nineteenth century, the professionalization of pharmacists paralleled that of physicians. By the turn of the century, as drug chemistry and the potential for addiction to certain drugs became more understood, the skills of pharmacists centered squarely on the knowledge and dispensing of medications instead of the earlier, more general skills of a hospital manager. Although no direct evidence links the professionalization of pharmacy to the Civil War, the separation of the types of stewards certainly focused the skills of apothecaries. Also, the Confederacy's shortage of medications and the subsequent investigations into the medicinal effectiveness of native plants and into opening new pharmaceutical laboratories prompted Southern apothecaries to develop their pharmaceutical skills. The distinction between the types of stewards was much more easily made at Chimborazo and other large hospitals whose patient load allowed for some individuals to be strictly designated as apothecary stewards and others to focus on the physical management of the wards. This concept was impractical in smaller facilities.

The importance of competent stewards and caring matrons in a hospital's staff cannot be overstated. They were the ones who made things work. Since they were in charge of the wards, kitchens, and laundry, they were the individuals who saw the problems that the patients saw and who had the ability to fix most things relating to the hospital's general environment. They heard the complaints and saw the problems before any other managers did. If the food was good, the clothes and bedding clean, and the general condition of the wards comfortable, then the rest of their jobs was made much easier. If problems arose in those general areas, then they were held accountable for the mismanagement of their staff and resources by both the surgeons and the patients. Along with their responsibilities in hospital management, they also had the authority to bring any problems they could not solve to the attention of the hospital's medical officers.

Although the positions of steward and matron did not focus on the medical care given to the patients, the nurses worked under the management of the stewards. Thus, if a problem arose involving the neglect or improper treatment of a patient, the steward could very well be in the middle of efforts to remedy the situation. All worked under the watchful eye of the matrons who could quickly find the surgeon-in-charge if necessary.

The combination of the steward and matrons worked very well. Each had his or her specific duties and responsibilities, but their goals overlapped enough to provide a check on each other. A good matron and good steward who worked well together as a team made their wards good places in which to recuperate. If one or the other was incompetent, the oversight of the good one would ensure that patient care did not suffer. If both were incompetent, problems arose but quickly came to the attention of the medical officer in charge. Thus, in the large hospitals many individuals looked out for the welfare of the patients. When mistakes were made by one, the others could often discover the problem and fix it before the situation deteriorated seriously.

Under the leadership of James Brown McCaw, all levels of Chimborazo's staff understood that their work would be judged by how it affected patient care. That criterion enabled the staff members to perform their jobs with the confidence that their efforts would be appreciated and their creativity encouraged as long as their work and ideas illustrated their devotion to improving patient care. The presence of the military hierarchy and the stability of the hospital's administration provided the necessary structure from which new ideas could develop. Because the hospital was a military institution, the staff could work toward its goals without the pressures of making a profit or satisfying a board of directors. As long as Chimborazo Hospital and others like it operated within Medical Department regulations, funded itself by using normal hospital rations, and provided good medical care, its physicians and staff had the freedom to provide that care in the best way they saw fit. Within that environment, the staff of Chimborazo worked to make their facility the best that it could possibly be. That effort, based on the dedication to patient care, was evident to Chimborazo's patients and made all the difference in their eyes as to the success of the hospital.

CHAPTER 4

The Patients

Chimborazo Hospital treated 77,889 patients during the Civil War. Each of those patients developed an opinion about the care he received while at the institution—an opinion that all shared with their families and friends through their letters and conversations. Although very few of these letters survive today for the historian to examine, it is possible to piece together the normal routine of the hospital and some of the patients' opinions and concerns about their lives while in the hospital. Receiving medical treatment is a very personal experience—one that is not quickly forgotten. The patients' perceptions about their hospital stay shaped the opinions about medical care, physicians, and hospitals that they carried with them for the rest of their lives. Their experiences at Chimborazo allowed them to see medicine in a positive light.

At the beginning of the war, virtually all soldiers objected to treatment in a hospital. A Union soldier wrote the following in an 1861 letter: "Our hospitals are so bad that our men fight against being sent to them. They will not go until they are compelled, and many brave it out and die in camp. I really believe they are more comfortable and better cared for in camp with their comrades, than in hospital."[1] This sentiment was commonly felt because many soldiers remembered the sick rooms of their past and believed that they had a better chance to recover from their wounds or disease if they could remain with friends or be sent home to family. A practical example of this sentiment can be seen in 1861 in Richmond after the First Battle of Manassas. Wounded Union captives were sent to the city's only hospital for care; the wounded Confederate soldiers were sent to numerous private homes in the city that opened their doors in the crisis.[2] Samuel Stout reported, "'Mothers in parting with their soldier boys would implore their Captains and Colonels to keep their precious children out of those horrid places, the hospitals,' and many officers promised to do so."[3] Necessity forced those officers to disregard those promises, and millions of men were sent to the hospitals for treatment and recovery. "For the first time a broad cross section of the male American population experienced the reality of institutional care," Charles Rosenberg wrote.[4] Numerous other Americans were exposed to hospitals through personal visits and the letters and stories of their friends and family members. A negative experience in a hospital would have reinforced their reluctance to go into one of the facilities. A positive experience prompted them to rethink their opinion.

Before reaching Chimborazo, a patient often first received medical care in a field hospital and then was transferred by ambulance or railroad to another hospital before being moved to Chimborazo. Most of Chimborazo's admissions were patients transferred in groups from field hospitals or general hospitals in other cities that needed to clear patients from their beds to prepare for an upcoming battle or campaign.

Chimborazo's records reveal that during the course of the war the hospital treated enlisted men from every state in the Confederacy. When Chimborazo opened, patients were commonly assigned to the division that had the most vacant beds. As the hospital system became more established, patients were often assigned to a division based on which state they called home. This process of assigning patients became formalized into policy in the middle of 1863 for the Richmond area. By that time Richmond's large general hospitals were established, and the surgeon general was finally in a position to close the smaller, less-suitable hospitals, which had been in service since their makeshift organization at the beginning of the war. William Carrington designated four of Chimborazo's divisions to serve patients from Virginia, Georgia, North Carolina, and Alabama. Chimborazo's fifth division, although designated to serve several states at different times, basically functioned as a miscellaneous division, admitting patients from many different states depending on the current needs. A review of Chimborazo's division patient registers reveals that this practice was followed fairly consistently, although there were some exceptions in every division.

The new organization of patients worked well for several reasons. First of all, supplies sent by specific states could find their way to the patients from that state much more easily than under the previous system. The new system also made it much easier for visitors and mail to find patients. When patients were intermingled, the correct and timely distribution of supplies and mail, critical to the health and morale of the patients, was almost impossible to accomplish. Nicholas A. Davis complained about the old system: "[T]he inconvenience and consequent suffering, no one can describe. If you had two friends wounded in the same fight, you would be fortunate, if in the city, you found them within two miles of each other."[5]

Keeping patients from the same state together also promoted a more peaceful atmosphere in the hospital's wards. Soldiers from different states could quickly become jealous of each other if they thought that one group was receiving special treatment or an unequal amount of food or supplies. For example, if half a ward received some extra food or supplies sent from its home state and the other half of the ward got nothing, the patients who went without protested, even if they understood why they had been denied the goods. This was the case especially when patients were from a poor state or one so far away that transportation problems interfered with their getting anything but the most basic goods.

The best example of this involved the patients from Maryland who had left their home state to fight for the Confederate cause. Many Confederate soldiers disliked these patients and were jealous of any goods they received. Since the state of Maryland had remained loyal to the Union, no supplies, food, or taxes were sent to the Confederate government. Thus, goods received by Confederate Marylanders were perceived as something taken away from soldiers and patients from the Confederate states. Although Marylanders seemed to be Pember's favorite patients, she did admit that they were "awkward customers," observing, "They were aware of how much they were entitled to, in food, surgical and medical attendance and general comfort, and were not afraid to speak loudly and openly of neglect."[6] Because of the general tension Marylanders caused when intermingled with patients from other states, McCaw allowed several wards in Chimborazo No. 2 to become Marylander wards exclusively. Pember stated that she was responsible for this change. Before appealing to McCaw, she had worked to convince Surgeon General Moore to set aside a small hospital for the Maryland soldiers, which he refused to do because of the expense. Some jealousy may have been present at Chimborazo when the Marylander wards were being prepared, because, as Pember noted, these wards were "freshly whitewashed, and adorned with cedar boughs."[7]

When a soldier arrived at Chimborazo, he normally first stopped at the central office to be admitted into the patient register and assigned to one of the hospital's five divisions. The surgeon-in-charge of the appropriate division then distributed the patients among his wards. The general practice was to keep these patients together in the same wards when possible in order to help morale and maintain the sense of familiarity. Medically, this usually did not cause a problem, because the transferred patients arrived at the hospitals in groups of "sick," "convalescent," "slightly wounded," and "wounded." Patients whose medical problems did not match those of the group they came with were assigned to or transferred to other wards or hospitals. For example, if a patient developed a contagious infection, he was transferred to an isolation ward treating that ailment so that he would not spread it to wounded patients who were otherwise doing well.

After the patients received their ward assignment, the clerk of the surgeon-in-charge gave each of them a bed ticket, which the patient presented to the head nurse or wardmaster of their ward. If a patient carried any personal belongings or valuables with him, those were given to the head nurse or ward master of each ward, who turned them over to the hospital's baggage master. A claim check, also referred to as a baggage ticket, was issued to the patient so that the items could be returned when the patient left Chimborazo.[8] Any arms or ammunition were turned over to the sergeant of the guard in return for another claim check. Upon admission to a ward, patients were given a complete examination by the assistant surgeon. The medical officer's diagnosis, instructions for treatment, and diet were written on the bed ticket, which was hung at the end of each patient's bed.

Beginning in 1863, all patients were bathed as soon as their condition permitted after admission. The bath served a "hygenic purpose." If the patients were ambulatory, they were ordered to the bathhouse on the hospital's grounds. Medical department regulations required all soldiers who had access to a bathhouse to bathe completely once a week and wash their hands and feet daily.[9] As an independent army post with a bathhouse, Chimborazo's patients fell under this regulation. Patients were also required to bathe before they were furloughed, transferred, or discharged from the hospital.[10]

The only exceptions to the routine admissions process occurred when the fighting drew close to Richmond and patients arrived at Chimborazo directly from the field, only four or five hours after being wounded. Then the hospital functioned more as a field hospital. In these cases, patients were treated first and officially admitted, if they needed long-term treatment, when time allowed. Phoebe Pember remembered this:

> About eight o'clock the slightly wounded began to straggle in with a bleeding hand, or contused arm or head, bound up in any convenient rag. . . . Few surgeons had remained in the hospital; the proximity to the field tempting them to join the ambulance committee, or ride to the scene of action; and the officer of the day, left in charge, naturally objected to my receiving a large body of suffering men with no arrangements made for their comfort, and but few in attendance.[11]

Pember insisted that she was not going to turn the men away without care; the medical officer relented and the men were attended to. It was during these periods of crisis that the matrons performed most of their nursing duties—in addition, of course, to their regular duties. The wounded patients got the beds of the convalescents, who were relegated to the floor or to tents hastily pitched around the hospital's perimeter. The situation remained taxing for both patients and staff until the fighting slowed enough to transfer some of the patients to other, less-crowded hospitals.

Patients quickly learned the routine of hospital life. The day began at Chimborazo with breakfast, which was served at 7:00 A.M. For all meals ambulatory patients ate in the hospital's dining room, while bedridden patients were fed by the nurses from the "matrons' table." At the beginning of the war, "Bakers bread, 3/4 pint of coffee, fish & Molasses" made up a typical breakfast.[12]

After breakfast, the assistant surgeons made rounds. Once rounds were completed, the matrons adjusted their diet rolls and made their rounds through the wards "for the purpose of speaking words of comfort to the sick, and remedying any apparent evils which had been overlooked or forgotten by the surgeons when going on their rounds."[13] At noon, the assistant surgeons reported to their surgeon-in-charge about the number of patients in their care and discussed any problems they were having in the wards. Dinner, the main meal of the day, was served at 2:00 P.M. McCaw ordered the following for the hospital's patients for dinner: "On Sundays and Wednesdays, Bacon; on all other days, Beef, fresh and corned, with ample allowance of vegetables: Irish and Sweet Potatoes, cabbage, Turnips, peas, stewed Peaches, apples & cold slaw daily for Dinner."[14]

At Chimborazo, another visit by the matrons usually occurred mid-afternoon although it was not required. Pember explained her motivation for afternoon rounds by saying, "[T]he fear that the nourishment furnished had not suited the tastes of the men . . . would again take me among them in the afternoon."[15] On their afternoon rounds, matrons became aware of any change in a patient's condition that might affect his supper, which was served at 6:00 P.M. Supper generally consisted only of a half-pint of coffee and biscuits.[16] Medications were given at 10:00 A.M., 2:00 P.M., 6:00 P.M., and bedtime.[17]

As patients became able, they were assigned to help with the maintenance and cleanliness of their wards. One such duty was the airing of patients' bedding. Sheets had to be aired; of the three sheets given to each patient, one was constantly either being aired or washed. In fair weather, regulations required that bedding filler and bedsacks be aired for at least two hours a day. The filling had to be completely replaced at least once a month. Patients might also be asked to help whitewash the wards, which was done several times each year, or dry-scrub the floors with sand, which was done weekly.[18] All of these tasks had to be done routinely, but nurses were generally too busy with sick patients to accomplish them by themselves.

Most of Chimborazo's patients were enlisted men, whom Pember described as "uneducated men, who had lived by the sweat of their brow."[19] Some evidently enjoyed hospital life so much that they worked diligently not to leave. These patients were commonly referred to as "hospital rats"—"would-be invalids who resisted being cured from a disinclination to field service. They were so called . . . from the difficulty of getting rid of either species."[20] Surgeon W. A. Davis described a good example of one of these hospital rats, a Private J. Hodnett from Alabama, whose original ailment, severe hemorrhoids, had disappeared:

> He has recently complained of multiform diseases of Genital, urinary, respiratory, circulatory, nervous, and digestive systems, and of fever intermittent. On careful examination no evidence of any of these diseases can be detected. Having fully satisfied myself that said Priv. Hodnett is a Malingerer, and being convinced that he is fit for duty, I have ordered him to rejoin his command.[21]

Another "hospital rat" who made it into Chimborazo's written record was Dennis Fitzgerald. Surgeon S. E. Habersham wrote to Brigadier General John Winder of this soldier. "[Fitzgerald] has been in this Hospital since its organization and has made constant application for a discharge. He has many complaints none of which are real, and finding it impossible to keep him from the bottle I returned him yesterday as fit for duty."[22]

Besides enlisted men, other categories of patients turned up at the Hospital on the Hill from time to time. One of these groups consisted of Confederate officers. Officers who needed medical treatment were usually assigned to private quarters as soon as their condition allowed. General Hospitals No. 4 and No. 10 were set aside for those officers in the Richmond area who needed treatment in a hospital setting.[23] However, even those hospitals could not escape the medical realities of the war. In mid-1864 Chimborazo received a number of officers as patients when General Hospital No. 4 was temporarily closed because of an outbreak of hospital gangrene at that facility. Interestingly enough, Pember reported, "I find in all the cases I have met with that [the officers] have been rougher than the men."[24]

Other patients who found themselves at Chimborazo were captured Union soldiers. The Confederate army preferred to keep the men in prisons or prison hospitals, which could be more easily guarded. The prison hospitals in Richmond were General Hospitals No. 13 and 18, both previously used as tobacco factories. The poor hygienic conditions of those buildings caused "great mortality and suffering" among the prisoners. In March 1864, Carrington wrote to General John Winder of the poor hygienic conditions of those buildings, explaining, "The great mortality and suffering among our prisoners has been a cause of constant anxiety and painful solicitude to me."[25] Carrington requested that the sick prisoners be transferred to other hospitals, such as Chimborazo. The letter seemed to cause the army to reconsider its previous position because three hundred prisoners were transferred to Chimborazo in April 1864—only a couple of weeks after the letter was sent. According to Carrington, "[Confederate] medical officers were directed to show the sick and wounded Federals all kindness and consideration, and to give them all the care possible under the circumstances."[26] In an interesting side note, about two weeks after the prisoners arrived, McCaw wrote Carrington to ask whether a paroled prisoner could act as a nurse in a Confederate hospital without violating his parole. Carrington said yes.[27]

Blacks suffering from illnesses formed another category of patients who found treatment at Chimborazo. This group included both enslaved and free black men who were employed by the Confederate government to work for the war effort. The initial attempt to admit blacks into Chimborazo occurred on March 14, 1862. W. A. Davis, surgeon-in-charge of Chimborazo No. 4, reported that an ambulance master named Peters had brought him "some negroes who had been employed in government work and were now on sick list, for whom he was seeking accommodation in Chimborazo Hospitals in accordance with an order from Genl. Winder. Said Peters produced no written order." After Davis refused to receive the patients, Peters "became pettish and dis-respectful" and Davis "dismissed him with a few curt remarks." Davis reminded McCaw that he had ordered Chimborazo No. 4 to prepare for a hundred soldiers, which had been done by readying new cots, beds and bedclothes, and new houses. He closed the letter by stating, "If I had received the negroes I should have been obliged to give to them these accommodations, to the exclusion of an equal number of soldiers and to the annoyance of a large number, as my hospital buildings are in close proximity. I have no isolated building fit for a negro ward."[28] Evidently, however, space was found at Chimborazo for the blacks, because on March 15, Surgeon L. Guild, an inspector of hospitals on Moore's staff, wrote to McCaw, directing "that the sick negroes, admitted into your hospital, be accommodated in a separate building—noting their number in your morning report under the column of 'Remarks.'"[29]

Later in the war the Surgeon General's Office found it necessary to increase the accommodations available for black patients. The office issued a circular to all medical directors at the end of 1864, stating, "The employment of negroes as teamsters & laborers, in the place of enlisted men, renders it necessary to provide special hospital accommodations for them." It directed the surgeons to reserve as many hospital tents or buildings necessary to treat these men.[30] By the time this circular was issued, Chimborazo had already treated several black patients. One example was I. C. Busch, who served with the Fifteenth Georgia Regiment. When he was admitted to Chimborazo, the clerk entered "colored" in the column of the patient register requesting the patient's rank. Busch was later returned to duty.[31]

A final category of patients—the rarest group—was that of civilians who for various reasons sought medical treatment at Chimborazo. These patients were recorded in the hospital's registers with "citizen" written in the space where a soldier's rank was usually entered. Most of these patients became seriously ill or injured while working for the Confederacy. It is interesting to note that one of the hospitals within Richmond's city limits would have been much more convenient for these civilian patients. L. S. Haggett, a citizen patient, was a Marylander working for the Confederate Quartermaster's Department; he was admitted to Chimborazo No. 4 in January 1864.[32] For some reason he and the other civilians chose Chimborazo.

A different—and unique—example of a citizen patient was a "Mrs. Daniells," a pregnant woman who was visiting her husband, a patient in Ward G of Chimborazo No. 2. While visiting, she went into labor and gave birth in the ward. The physician ordered that the new mother be moved to an empty ward and given tea and toast. The ladies of Richmond provided her with a ticket home to West Virginia and some clothing for herself and her baby. Sadly, the woman cashed in her ticket and deserted the infant at the railroad station. As soon as was possible, the father was granted a short furlough so that he could take the baby home to his relatives.[33]

With the wide variety of patients and staff who lived at Chimborazo, the hospital passed regulations restricting patients' behavior to keep order in its wards. No copies of Chimborazo's regulations for patients' behavior survive, but available records from Winder Hospital and other large general hospitals are very similar to one another and can be used to approximate those at Chimborazo. Rev. Nicholas A. Davis, a chaplain with the Fourth Texas Regiment, commented in 1863, "The rules and regulations of the Hospitals have . . . been systematized and adapted to the comfort of the patients, as well as to the convenience of their friends, who come to look after, and do offices of kindness for them."[34]

Some regulations reinforced the idea of the authority of the hospital's staff. Medical officers, nurses, wardmasters, and other staff were to be obeyed and treated respectfully. Disrespect on the part of patients or unkindness or neglect on the part of staff was to be reported to the assistant surgeon or surgeon-in-charge. Other regulations restricted patients' movements. Patients had to be at their own beds during the assistant surgeon's rounds and could not leave the hospital's grounds without a written pass, signed by the surgeon-in-charge of their hospital. Still other regulations prohibited improper behavior so as to improve the overall environment of the hospital and its wards. Besides stating that no "disorderly conduct" was tolerated, specific regulations forbade loud talking, "profane swearing," smoking tobacco, unprescribed liquor, and "loafing about the Clerk's office and Drug store." Some hospitals banned chewing tobacco in the wards, while others allowed chewing tobacco as long as the patients used the spitoons provided and did not spit on the walls or floors. Regulations similar to those in military hospitals had been in place in civilian hospitals for years, but enforcement was a common problem. Regulations seemed more understandable in a military situation, in which rules of conduct always applied.[35]

Chimborazo's guard enforced the hospital's regulations, as well as the military regulations that governed behavior at Chimborazo in general. Patients violating the regulations or stealing hospital supplies could be arrested and confined to the guard house. The presence of a guard, routine on army posts but not at hospitals, made Chimborazo Hospital different from many others at the beginning of the war. The absence of a guard unit at Gordon Hospital in Nashville early in the war permitted patients to wander off from the facility unchecked.[36] The enforcement of the regulations by an armed guard allowed order to rule on the hospital's grounds.

The guard unit at Chimborazo was implemented in July 1862 when one non-commissioned officer and twelve men were sent to the hospital for that purpose.[37] I. B. Yarrington, described in correspondence as "a reliable man," served as the sergeant of the guard at Chimborazo during much of the war. He was paid $2.50 per day for his services.[38] As supplies grew more scarce the demand for reliable guards increased, prompting Moore to instruct, "Soldiers who have lost their hand or arm and are otherwise healthy, but are incompetent to perform clerical duty, can, in the use of a pistol, act as efficient guards for Hospitals and Purveying Depots. The majority of the guard can be composed of such men."[39]

By mid-1864 the hospital's guard had grown to twenty-six men and evidently was still understaffed. When Carrington requested that ten guards be sent from the hospital for temporary duty in Richmond, McCaw replied that the twenty new guards who had been assigned to the hospital had never showed up. "If we send 10 men to Surg Gravatt we would have but two reliefs."[40] In August, 1864, McCaw wrote to Carrington asking for more men: "The sergeant of the Guard has only 18 men—we require not less than fifty—38 deficiency."[41]

As the war continued and the army needed all healthy men for its ranks, it became harder for McCaw to maintain an adequate guard. In January 1864, Carrington ordered McCaw to "discharge from the guard all employed men, without delay, and direct them to report at the Enrolling Office. . . . Other guards will be furnished from the detailed soldiers if required." McCaw complied, but "respectfully suggested that Sergt Yarrington should not be discharged; . . . There would be no head left & his guardhouse would be under no control." Carrington agreed that Yarrington should be retained. The rest of the guard unit was replaced by some detailed men sent to Chimborazo to act as guards; the guard was rounded out by convalescent patients who were sent to the guardhouse for duty as needed.[42]

Although life in a Confederate hospital was very different from the men's normal lives, every attempt was made to keep the patients at Chimborazo comfortable and connected to the rest of society. Unlike civilian patients in antebellum hospitals, patients in Confederate hospitals were valued. Most were productive members of society who had enlisted in the army to fight for their states, their beliefs, and their way of life. As soon as they recuperated, they would be transferred back to the fighting and continue their contributions to the Confederate war effort, just like every surgeon, steward, and matron at Chimborazo. To recuperate quickly and then to fight effectively, the patients had to keep their morale up and their connection to the society they fought for firm.

In part this was accomplished through letters from home. Mail was delivered and picked up daily, and patients were encouraged to write letters to their families and friends. If a patient was illiterate or unable to write and had no friends in the same ward who could help him, his matron could read his mail to him and then write down his response to be mailed.

Taking part in political elections also contributed to the sense of connection to normal life. Recognizing that the patients were also voting citizens, arrangements were made in 1864 so that patients could vote in the elections for senators and other Confederate government officials while at Chimborazo.[43]

Various services were also provided to the patients. Barbers and dentists came to the hospital weekly to provide their services to the patients. Some hospitals set up libraries for their patients; others purchased newspapers for the patients using the hospital fund.[44] Chaplains were hired to provide for the spiritual needs of the hospital's patients. The chaplains were charged with the responsibility to "take a sufficient interest in the spiritual welfare of the soldiers and furnish him with the necessary books, etc. to secure his attention and interest."[45] The main chaplain at Chimborazo was Rev. Patterson, who had immigrated to the United States from Greece as an adult. He was described as "a very valuable officer."[46]

Celebrating the holidays was another way that patients could retain some semblance of regular life. Christmas Day was the major holiday observed at Chimborazo. No extra monies could be taken from any official source to fund a celebration, so the hospital's matrons had to be creative in making this holiday special for their patients. In 1863 Pember and Chimborazo's other matrons raised money for a special Christmas dinner by "condemning old comforts and blankets and having them sold, adding all donations received from private individuals."[47] They made enough money to be able to give each patient some turkey and oysters, a slice of cake, and some eggnog. When McCaw saw the meal and inquired how such a feat had been accomplished, Pember explained it to him. "[H]e laughed heartily," she recalled, "and said I was a monstrous humbug, but seemed very much pleased."[48] When Christmas arrived the following year, times were much harder. The festivities depended on the women of Richmond, who drove out in their carriages with baskets of delicacies for the men.[49]

However much the men enjoyed and appreciated special events such as Christmas, too much time passed between special events and letters from home for the patients at Chimborazo not to grow bored. Many sick or convalescent patients were too ill to rejoin their regiments in the field but also too strong to be content to lie peacefully in their beds all day. In her memoirs, Phoebe Pember described several ways that her patients kept themselves occupied. Playing cards—"the greatest comfort to alleviate the tedium of their sick life"—was an especially popular pastime. Pember reported that the decks were used so often that the cards quickly became dirty and their corners grew worn. To solve this problem, the soldiers learned to round the corners of their cards—an idea they took from a set of Bibles donated from England.[50]

Craftsmanship also became an outlet for the patients' energies. Pember remembered some examples:

> The ingenuity of the men was wonderful in making toys and trifles, and a great deal of mechanical talent was developed by the enforced inaction of hospital life. Every ward had its draught-board and draughtsmen cut out of hard wood and stained with vegetable dies [*sic*], and sometimes chessmen would be cut out with a common knife, in such ornamentation that they would not have disgraced a drawing-room. One man carved pipes from ivy root, with exquisitely-cut shields on the bowls, bearing the arms of different states, and their mottoes. He would charge and easily get a hundred and fifty dollars for a pipe.[51]

McCaw also recognized this craftsmanship by recovering patients. In October 1862 he wrote to the medical director with the idea that talented patients, such as tailors and cobblers, could be put to work making shoes and other items if the army would supply them with the necessary leather and other supplies.[52] Existing hospital records make no mention of action being taken on this suggestion. However, in September 1863 the surgeon general requested information from McCaw about Chimborazo patients who were coopers by trade.[53]

Another way in which the men fought the monotony of hospital life was by altering the clothing the army issued to them. In one example of this, patients made changes to some unpopular canvas shoes they had received from the quartermaster. "[T]here was a loud dissatisfaction expressed in constant grumbling, till some original genius dyed the whitish tops by the liberal application of poke berries," Pember recalled. "He was the Brummel of the day, and for many months crimson shoes were the rage, and long rows of unshod men would sit under the eaves of the wards, all diligently employed in the same labor and up to their elbows in red juice."[54] After the appeal of dyed shoes faded, patients next focused on "button-mania."

Less savory activities were also available to those ambulatory patients who could obtain hard-to-get temporary passes into Richmond. In July 1864 the *Richmond*

Daily Whig reported that Chimborazo patients J. M. Boykin and R. Holesforth were two of three clients who were dragged out of a prostitution establishment during a police raid.[55]

When not busy with other activities, patients would occupy themselves with conversation. Since many patients in a ward were from the same regiment or state, they often had shared experiences in camp or on the battlefield that they would repeatedly relive while recuperating. Pember reported, "The wounded wards would be noisily gay with singing, laughing, fighting battles o'er and o'er again, and playfully chaffing each other by decrying the troops from different states, each man applauding his own."[56]

Another subject of conversation was the hospital's rodent population. The rats seemed to be especially troublesome, whatever the season or the weather. These clever vermin effectively eluded attempts to kill or capture them. As Pember explained, "Hunger had educated their minds and sharpened their reasoning faculties."[57] At night the rats would eat poultices applied to the sick patients and drag off the bran-stuffed pads given to the wounded to support their injured limbs. Although troublesome, most patients seemed to find the rats' activities amusing. "The men related wonderful rat-stories," noted Pember.[58] Evidently, rats were a common problem for hospitals everywhere. Matron Emily Mason, who served at Winder Hospital, controlled a crisis by reminding her patients of her willingness to stew the rats they had caught when the cook refused.[59]

Of course, of all the ways to pass the time, nothing could compare with a visit from home. Before the Civil War, hospitals rarely had visitors. The nature of the patients during the war made visitors to hospitals common, especially if the hospital treated patients from that region. Chimborazo encouraged visitors for its patients and made arrangements so that the visitors could reach the facility via road or boat. The boat, the most common means of transportation for day visitors who did not have a personal carriage, ran from the State Depot on Shockoe Slip in Richmond to Chimborazo twice daily for a moderate price. The State Depot also provided visitors with access to an updated, alphabetically arranged directory of the hospital's patients. Since Chimborazo cared for most of Virginia's sick and wounded in the Richmond area, the hospital's patients had many visitors. Pember's division, which consisted chiefly of soldiers from Virginia and Maryland, received the majority of the visitors. She wrote, "[T]he nearness of the homes of the former entailed upon me an increase of care in the shape of wives, sisters, cousins, aunts, and whole families, including the historic baby at the breast. They came in troops, and hard as it was to know how to dispose of them, it was harder to send them away."[60]

Although some visitors abided by the rules set up by the hospital, others, upset by the fact that their loved ones had to be kept in a hospital when they were so close to home, tested the limits of the hospital's staff. Many practical problems arose in the presence of visitors. Often several people would come at the same time to see a particular patient. If a particularly large group came, the issue of where to put all of them during their visit could become a problem. Also, since the trip out to Chimborazo was normally an all-day affair for visitors, meal times were sometimes difficult. Some families brought food with them. Sometimes the food had been cooked in advance; at other times the families brought the ingredients, expecting a stove or fire to be available. Others expected the hospital to provide them with at least a light snack while the patients ate. Matrons and stewards could not allow this, especially when food supplies for the patients were at times so limited. Of course, any "hospital food" that was provided to patients was frequently criticized by visitors and patients alike. As a result, visitors often brought foods for their patients to eat. Many times these foods were favorites of the patient but could not be allowed because their heavy or rich nature went against doctor's orders. This decision inevitably upset the visitors, who frequently fed their goodies to the patient while the medical staff was not paying attention.[61]

Surgeon Samuel Stout, while setting up his first hospital for a regiment from Tennessee, experienced problems with visitors who questioned the medical treatment for measles being given to the patients. As Stout's biographer noted, "They supposed that the patient should be kept warm with hot tea and alcoholic beverages in an unventilated room to make the measles break out. Despite the pleasant weather, they thought that staying in a tent would be fatal to the patient."[62] Stout had no choice but to keep the patients in the tents and try to keep out the alcohol that visitors would smuggle in.

Another common problem surfaced when visitors refused to go home. Pember recalled her frustration when a family visiting a patient who was recovering from typhoid fever "marched on me *en masse* at ten o'clock at night, with a requisition from the boldest for sleeping quarters. The steward was summoned, and said 'he didn't keep a hotel,' so in a weak moment of pity for their desolate state, I imprudently housed them in my laundry. They entrenched themselves there for six days."[63] The wife of this patient refused to leave the hospital even when her husband was released to be returned to duty, firmly believing that he would be wounded and returned to Chimborazo, which he was.

Still another dilemma occurred when the visitors appeared destitute and requested help or a job from the medical staff. Surgeon W. A. Davis wrote to McCaw about the wife of Private A. Myers, an Alabama infantryman who was a patient under his care in Chimborazo No. 4. Mrs. Myers came to Chimborazo with three small children in a government ambulance, saying that she had previously worked for the government as a laundress and had been sent to work at Chimborazo when her husband was taken there. Davis took pity on the woman, who said she had no resources in Richmond and appeared "very destitute [*sic*]"; thus, he provided for her and her children from his private means. Davis, knowing it was "not fit for her to remain in this hospital," asked McCaw what to do. No response was recorded.[64]

Surprisingly, there are no records of a patient's family adamantly insisting that he be sent home with them. One reason was probably the military nature of the situation. The patient remained a Confederate soldier even when he was in a hospital. To leave against the orders of the physicians would constitute desertion. Also, since the patient was a soldier, the government was paying for his medical care—an expense that could be extreme for the family of a seriously sick or injured patient who returned home. Another factor was the quality of medical care that he received in the hospital. Although a big part of treatment was keeping the patient comfortable, medications, specialty splints, and other medical items were not readily available to most Southerners. The shortage of medicine in the South made it difficult for civilians to gain access to morphine and other strong painkillers, which were mainly produced by Confederate Medical Department laboratories. Having the hospital matrons and friends of the soldier close by may also have eased a family's anxieties about leaving their husband or son in the care of the hospital.

At the beginning of the war, it was relatively easy for a patient to obtain a furlough home or a transfer into private quarters until he recuperated sufficiently to rejoin his unit. The two options were of a different nature, but both allowed the patient to move outside the hospital to a more comfortable setting and opened up another hospital bed for a critically ill patient who needed constant medical care. These practices, which agreed with the commonly held view that the domestic setting was best for the sick, helped to alleviate the shortage of hospital beds that hampered the Medical Department in 1861 and 1862.

There were available means for recuperating patients to leave Chimborazo. An examining board, made up of the higher ranking medical officers of the hospital, determined whether a patient qualified for a furlough or a medical discharge or whether he should be put on a detail. The following regulations submitted by McCaw and published in the *Richmond Daily Whig* clarified for the public what requirements had to be met for patients to leave Chimborazo on those terms: "Soldiers found unfit for any duty will be recommended for Discharge. If useful in other Departments, and unable to perform field service, a detail will be recommended. The Board will grant Furloughs when the patient will not be fit for duty in thirty days, and can bear transportation, provided his home is not within the enemy's lines."[65]

Furloughs were granted to patients whose medical situation had improved to the point that they mainly needed time to recuperate. Instead of recuperating in the hospital, a furlough sent the patient home for a short time to regain his strength, which saved the Confederacy the cost of additional time in the hospital and thrilled the men. Pember aptly described the furlough as the "El Dorado to the sick soldier."[66] The timing of the board's examination was critical. If the board determined that the patient would need more time than that to recover, he was considered a convalescent patient and either moved into a convalescent ward or to the "Soldiers' Home," a convalescent hospital in the area. If he needed only a week or so—not enough time to travel home to his family in most cases—he was moved into a convalescent ward and reexamined shortly afterward to determine when he could return to duty.

Even when a furlough had been granted, the soldier still had to wait for transportation home to be arranged. Just before the patient was ready to depart the hospital, the officer of the day examined him one last time to ensure that he was indeed healthy enough to leave. Surgeon Habersham, in charge of Chimborazo No. 2, ordered, "If the soldier furloughed should be deemed too weak or physically unable to bear the journey the Officer will detain him until he is and report his case on his Morning Report."[67] The case of Private Finley P. Curtis of the First North Carolina Infantry provided proof that this practice occurred. After a month-long stay at Chimborazo, Curtis was granted a furlough. "Father came to take me home, but not until I was safe from relapse would the physicians allow me to depart," he recalled.[68] To help patients as they made their way home, the Confederate government established a number of "way hospitals" along major railways to help soldiers who had been furloughed or discharged because of sickness or wounds.[69]

Furloughs became harder to obtain after December 1862, when the medical department issued a circular that stated, "Applications for furlough will hereafter only be made, when the changes contemplated are absolutely necessary for the convalescence of the Patient, and this fact will be stated in each application."[70] As the size of the army shrank, the number of furloughed patients decreased even further. Many army field commanders protested strongly against medical furloughs, arguing that many soldiers never returned to the ranks afterwards. However, they did continue to be granted throughout the war. With regard to Chimborazo, Carrington instructed McCaw in 1864 that the hospital's examining board be more lenient in issuing furloughs: "With so many under your charge, several hundred should be furloughed daily."[71]

Another major reason for the increased difficulty in getting a furlough toward the end of the war was the crippled transportation system in the South. If the government could not provide transportation to and from a furlough, medical officers were ordered not to grant it. An example of this occurred in February 1865. Carrington wrote to McCaw with the following directions: "[G]ive no furloughs to sick and wounded men to go beyond Columbia, So Carolina, until further orders. Transportation cannot be furnished further."[72] If a patient's home was behind enemy lines, it would be impossible for him to go home and then return to his regiment. One way that the Confederate government tried to improve this situation was by encouraging Virginians living near major hospitals and railroads to open their homes to these men. After a Richmond newspaper ran a story in June 1864 expressing the need for such hospitality, Carrington directed McCaw to examine and "forward lists to this Office of such men in the Hospital under your charge as are embraced in this class, in order that persons responding to this notice may be supplied without delay with as many as they are willing to receive."[73]

Being allowed to go into private quarters was the other non-hospital option for a patient's medical care. Surgeons had the authority to assign patients to private quarters if they met certain criteria. The following appeared in Chimborazo's statement of "Rules for the Government of Patients in Private Quarters": "No patient is allowed to go to private Quarters whose case can be treated to more advantage at the Hospital—who is known to be not trustworthy from previous experience or who is under charge for any Military offence [*sic*]."[74] Both officers and enlisted men could qualify but the economic situation of the patient was definitely considered, since the patient in private quarters had to be able to pay for his own lodging, food, and nursing care.[75] Any required medications would be ordered by the attending physician and then filled by a pharmacist, who would be paid by the medical purveyor.[76]

Every patient in private quarters remained under the supervision of a medical officer. When the patient was allowed to leave the hospital, he was assigned to a physician who was required to examine the patient on a regular basis. All patients in private quarters assigned to Chimborazo's physicians had to report to the hospital on Saturdays between 9:00 A.M. and 12:00 noon. If a patient was not able to come to the hospital, the assigned physician examined him at the patient's location sometime between 3:00 P.M. on Saturday and 12:00 noon on Sunday. Chimborazo's regulations read, "All patients who do not report sanctually in person when they are able will have their permits irrevocably withdrawn."[77] The penalty for not reporting was strengthened in June 1864. Carrington ordered surgeons to report patients who had not shown up for their weekly visit to the Confederate police at the Provost Marshall's Office, who would then arrest the patient and return him to the hospital.[78] Because of the "great abuses" in the system, the assistant adjutant general of the Medical Department began to provide all patients who were allowed to remain in private quarters with an official pass. Without this pass, they would be reported as being absent without leave.[79]

Although diligent supervision of patients in private quarters was expected, there are indications that the system was less than perfect. After realizing how many men from Chimborazo were in private quarters, Carrington responded in a letter to McCaw:

> The very large number of men in Private Quarters from Chimborazo
> Hospl [*sic*] cannot have the supervision of the Surgeons in charge of
> the Divisions. I direct that each one of them be examined by a Medical
> Officer of the Hospl within the next week. Those fit for detail will be
> sent to their regiments for examination for such detail; those who
> are injured by want of restraint will be readmitted into the Hospital.
> Those who require a change of air or scenery will be recommended for

transfer to other Hospls or furloughed. The men in future who apply for transfer to private quarters I prefer should be transferred to the Confederate Hospitals in this city to which they live nearest."[60]

By the end of 1864, very few of Chimborazo's patients were assigned to private quarters. For one thing, food and lodging in Richmond were so outrageously expensive by late in the war that very few enlisted patients could afford them. If patients could afford the cost, surgeons were instructed not to so indulge any patient who had ever abused the privilege or who might not closely follow the medical orders prescribed. Soldiers fit for duty in the hospital or on a detail and those who could qualify for a furlough were also excluded from private quarters.[81]

Transfers from Chimborazo to another hospital could be ordered if the situation required it. Developing smallpox, for example, ensured a quick transfer. If the patient was at Chimborazo or in the Richmond area, he was sent to Howard's Grove Hospital. Toward the end of the war, patients with certain orthopedic problems were transferred to Robertson Hospital in Richmond to be treated by Richmond's specialist in that area. Transfers to state hospitals could also be granted "where persons have fathers, mothers, or wives who come for them to go short distances . . . to Hospitals near home and do not ask for transportation."[82] Finally, transfers of groups of patients routinely occurred when a battle was imminent and the hospitals closest to the fighting needed room for patients fresh from the battlefield. Chimborazo usually transferred its patients to hospitals at Danville, Staunton, and Farmville, Virginia—all of which had been established because of their easy access to the railroad.

Desertion from Chimborazo did occur but not very often. W. A. Davis, the surgeon-in-charge of Chimborazo No. 4, explained to McCaw, "My men generally manifest an aversion to going to the Soldiers home, as preliminary to a return to duty."[83] Davis believed that when the men received orders to the Soldiers' Home, many went home instead, intending to rejoin their units in the field when they had recuperated fully.

Death was the only other way for a patient to leave Chimborazo Hospital. The first patient to die at Chimborazo was Private S. Cono of Georgia, who succumbed to typhoid fever on October 25, 1861.[84] When a patient died, the officer of the day was notified to examine the body and sign the death certificate. The patient's name was entered in his division's death register. Each of the hospital's five divisions had its own deadhouse. When a soldier died, the steward placed the person's name, rank, company, and regiment, "pinned or sewed on securely," on the body's breast before it was moved from the ward to the deadhouse.[85] The bodies were then properly dressed before being sent to the nearest cemetery for interment.

Oakwood Cemetery, located three-fourths of a mile northeast of Chimborazo, was the normal burial place for the hospital's dead. The small country cemetery had rarely been used before the war, but that changed during the war, when Oakwood received more than sixteen thousand Confederate soldiers to its grounds because of its close proximity to Chimborazo and Howard's Grove Hospitals. J. Boulware, a hospital steward with the Sixth South Carolina Volunteers, provided a description of this cemetery in his journal: "The situation is well chosen and beautifully laid out and planted with trees of various kinds. It covers ten or twelve acres. Most of the graves seem fresh. Very few have marble headstones, yet all have boards with name, company, regiment and state. So by referring to the keeper's book, anyone may find the grave of relative or friend."[86]

It is important to realize that Howard's Grove Hospital also used this cemetery, because some past writers have based their calculations of Chimborazo's mortality rate on the number of admissions into the cemetery during the war. When Howard's Grove's use of Oakwood is not taken into account, the mortality rate at Chimborazo appears to be over 20 percent, instead of 11.29 percent. One should remember, too, that Howard's Grove Hospital served as the area's smallpox hospital. Also, as Ernest B. Furgurson wrote in his book *Ashes of Glory,* the other major cemetery in Richmond, Hollywood Cemetery, had become full by mid-1862. Furgurson continued, "[W]orkers started burying soldiers beyond its boundary, on land near the city. This practice was halted by the city's health board."[87] Thus, any calculations for mortality rates based only on numbers of bodies in Oakwood Cemetery can in no way be considered accurate.

A few of Chimborazo's dead were sent to their homes at the request of their families, who paid for the cost of transportation. A very few were buried in other cemeteries in the area. Pember documented one such case—"a Marylander who begged to be buried apart from the crowd." She took his body in her ambulance to Hollywood Cemetery on the other side of Richmond, about five miles from Chimborazo. She would have rented a hearse, but Richmond was under attack, forcing her to use her ambulance to transport the coffin.[88]

Since most patients could not leave the hospital until their health improved, they spent time voicing complaints about problems or injustices and trying to alleviate those difficulties. The patients at Chimborazo realized that the medical staff listened to their complaints. In December 1862 patients wrote the following letter to McCaw:

> We the sick and afflicted of the Hospital having become tired of the manner in which Mr. Miller, the PostMaster casts out the mail, do earnestly request you to remove him and put some one in the office who is competent to discharge the duties of the office satisfactory to the patrons of the office. Our objection to him is this that he miscalls more than half of the letters, and it takes him four times as long as it ought to call out the mail and when he calls a letter, he holds it up in

the air, sometimes for minutes before he will deliver it to the person it is for. Your attention to this matter will greatly oblige the inmates of Chimborazo.[89]

This complaint about the practices of the postmaster is significant in several ways. First of all, the patients evidently believed that McCaw might well do something to remedy the situation, or else they would not have called his attention to it. Also, if they trusted McCaw to change a relatively minor problem, they must have felt comfortable about contacting him if a major difficulty arose.

Most patient complaints were taken seriously by medical officers. If a patient's request was not honored by an assistant surgeon or other medical officer at his hospital, the patient wrote home about the situation, and his concerns sometimes reached the medical director or surgeon general via letters from the patient's family or influential friends. When complaints reached Carrington about patients at Chimborazo not being able to have a haircut or shave, he instructed McCaw "to employ a Barber, with the pay of Nurse, for each one or more divisions . . . as may be necessary."[90] Another example concerned food. Convalescents in the Fourth Alabama Division wrote home about bad food. The families passed on the complaints to Alabama officials, who wrote to Carrington. In response, Carrington requested a daily written report from the officer of the day in each division about the condition of the food and dining rooms. He also requested a surprise inspection by McCaw.[91]

Although patients had various complaints, Chimborazo Hospital was recognized as one of the best military hospitals in the South. Historical records show several cases where individuals chose to stay at the Hospital on the Hill when they could have gone to another. When Philip Whitlock, a private from the Twelfth Virginia Infantry, became sick, he was transferred to Chimborazo "'through the activity and intercidence' of his brother and brother-in-law."[92] Another example was Sergeant J. L. Wagner, who had been admitted in November 1863 while still recuperating from a gunshot wound to the abdomen that he had received at Gettysburg. Surgeon W. A. Davis wrote, "He will be unfit for duty for next fifty days—but having no accessible home wishes to remain in Hospital."[93] Davis requested a permit for Wagner so that he could walk about the city while recuperating at the hospital.

Most patients endured the situation at Chimborazo just as they endured life in camp—by trying to make the best of a bad situation. They realized that certain problems were unavoidable. The lack of supplies plagued the entire Confederacy. Some sicknesses could not be cured, no matter how talented or dedicated the medical staff might be. And, no matter how hard the staff of the hospital tried to improve the situation, the nature of any hospital is that it houses people who are sick or hurt. In the mid-nineteenth century, before the value of cleanliness was truly understood in medical terms, hospitals were not places where people wanted to be. Even today, with private rooms and cutting-edge medical technology, both patients and visitors dislike hospitals. However, the hospital setting at Chimborazo was tolerable enough that people began to see the hospitals in general as an option when they needed medical treatment. The action of one soldier from Virginia documents this. The condition of Private J. W. S. Land grew worse while at home on a furlough; he returned to Chimborazo one week early and was readmitted for treatment.[94] The hospital, with all its problems and unpleasantness, had proven itself in the mind of Private Land as a place where he could get better medical care than he could at home. Patients left the hospital remembering not just the problems but also the possibilities.

One positive aspect of Chimborazo was the patients' ability to affect the medical treatment they received there. Patients could refuse to consent to an operation. A private from Alabama named Hodnett, who was assigned to Chimborazo No. 4, refused to allow a surgeon to perform a needed operation. After an unsuccessful appeal to the Board of Surgeons at Chimborazo, the patient continued to refuse the operation and asked McCaw that he be allowed to return to duty in his present condition. McCaw wrote to Carrington, who in turn wrote to Moore, to get a final decision on the matter. Moore replied that the patient would be compelled to have the surgery but that he would allow Private Hodnett to be transferred first to the General Hospital in Montgomery, Alabama.[95] In a less serious case, a starch bandage was removed from a patient at Chimborazo No. 2 at the patient's request because it was uncomfortable.[96]

The most positive memories that many patients took with them from Chimborazo involved the people they met and came to know. Private M. T. Leadbetter, who was admitted to Chimborazo on June 29, 1862, wrote, "The servants waited on me nicely, and brought me plenty to eat. My ward master was a whole-souled and jolly kind of a fellow. I became very much attached to him."[97] Another example came from Corporal William E. Traher of Company E, Sixth Louisiana Infantry, who was admitted to Chimborazo in August 1863 for diabetes. While convalescing at the hospital, he became an assistant clerk in McCaw's office and was put in charge of the payroll for the patients. After returning to his unit in the field several months later, Traher was wounded and taken to the Lady's Relief Hospital in Lynchburg, which transferred him with other patients to the "larger and better hospital in Richmond" on May 12. Traher wrote, "My heart was in a great flutter of joy, in the prospect of being in Richmond again. All my best friends were there, and I longed to meet them." Once again at Chimborazo, "[i]t was pleasant indeed, when I found myself in the same division . . . occupied a year before, with the same surgeon . . . and the same Supt. and assistants."[98]

Through patients' experiences, their perception of hospitals changed. Confederate surgeon Spencer Welch commented in a letter to his wife: "Last year when a soldier was sent to a hospital he was expected to die, but all who come from the hospitals in Richmond now are highly pleased with the treatment they received."[99] By 1863 one Richmond visitor observed "that the hospital accommodations in and around the capital were 'most perfect and ample for such of our sick and wounded soldiers as may be sent to this point.'"[100] More evidence for the improvement can be seen in a Richmond newspaper's comment that the medical staff was "fast approaching perfection in the systematic arrangement of the various hospitals in and around the city."[101] Such changes occurred in both the North and the South. General U. S. Grant wrote to Surgeon General William Hammond in 1863, "It is a great question whether one person in ten could be so well taken care of at home as in the army here."[102] Louisa May Alcott reported another example in her popular book, *Hospital Sketches* (1863), which recounted her experiences as a volunteer nurse. Upon leaving her hospital, one of her patients said, "We're off, ma'am, and I'm powerful sorry, for I'd no idea a 'orspittle was such a jolly place. Hope I'll git another ball somewheres else, so I'll come back, and be took care of again."[103]

A sense of camaraderie had developed at Chimborazo, as well as a sense of trust—trust that the people who worked at the hospital saw the patients as individuals worthy of respect. Once this level of trust had been achieved, the view of hospitals as a place where only society's worthless went to die had been broken. The patients at Chimborazo and the visitors who came to see them began to view hospitals in a new light. Although people still considered the home setting preferable, as it is today, they also realized that medical care in a large institutional setting could work effectively. The shifts in attitude of the public and the medical community with regard to the treatment of patients in large hospitals was critical to the development of the modern civilian hospital system.

CHAPTER **5**

Supplies

The task of obtaining sufficient supplies for Chimborazo Hospital required the full time efforts of many individuals. Starting from scratch in 1861, the officials at the facility had to provide food, clothing, shelter, and medical care for thousands of patients and a large staff. The ability to obtain supplies was critically important for the welfare and morale of Chimborazo's inhabitants. Patients may not have understood specific medical treatments or practices, but they were very astute about their needs for clean clothing, warm bedding, comfortable surroundings, and good food. The importance of those items is intensified for the person who is sick or wounded and separated from family and friends. The hospital's staff could not have effectively treated the patients without adequate supplies. Food, clothing, shelter, and medical supplies were all essential elements of patient care at Chimborazo. If any one of them was not available or was inadequate, then patients would not recover as quickly as possible and the morale of the hospital's staff would suffer. A lack of supplies would overshadow all other concerns, diverting attention away from the quality of care and environment at Chimborazo and severely diminishing the perception of the hospital as an effective institution. The talent of Chimborazo's personnel and the administration's creative approach to the bureaucracy and regulations of the Confederate army made it possible for the hospital to obtain the necessary supplies until the very end of the war, thus illustrating another reason why Chimborazo was widely recognized as an excellent Confederate hospital.

The shortage of supplies that faced the Confederacy is widely recognized. Chimborazo was not immune to this problem, especially since it was located just outside of Richmond—one of the cities hardest hit by the shortages. When looking at the hospital's surviving records, especially those from 1864 and 1865, one cannot help but be struck by the shortages encountered. At first glance, it appears that the patients of Chimborazo were upset by the apparent lack of supplies, perhaps blaming the large size of the institution or hospitals in general for their inability to obtain the necessary amounts of food, fuel, and other materials. However, to understand the supplies situation fully, one must recognize the difficulties faced by all Confederate soldiers and citizens in obtaining supplies. As the Union blockade tightened, many goods that were commonly used in the early years of the war simply became unobtainable. The prices of many other items rose so dramatically that only the wealthiest Southerners could afford them.

The crowded condition of Richmond and the inordinate amount of fighting that occurred in northern Virginia exacerbated the region's supplies problems. In his book on Confederate Richmond, Ernest B. Furgurson stated, "Richmond was by far the most expensive, corrupt, overcrowded, and crime-ridden city in the Confederacy. At one point prices in Columbia, South Carolina, were only a fiftieth of those in Richmond; cane syrup selling for $1 a gallon in rural Georgia was $50 in the capital."[1]

Thus, the amazing thing about the supplies situation at Chimborazo was not the shortages that occurred there but instead the hospital staff's ability to obtain supplies until the last months of the war. The main reason for Chimborazo's success in this area was McCaw's determination, tenacity, and creativity in making his hospital as self-sufficient as possible. Although regulations required him to work through the appropriate military departments responsible for obtaining food and supplies, McCaw refused to use the regulations as an excuse to relieve himself from the responsibility of providing for his patients and staff. If McCaw discovered that the commissary or quartermaster's departments had supplies in local warehouses that his hospital needed, he immediately contacted the appropriate officers, filled out the paperwork, and sent Chimborazo's wagons for the goods. The timely and diligent action of Chimborazo's staff allowed their hospital to obtain supplies when others failed. More important, from the beginning of McCaw's tenure at the hospital, he tested the flexibility of the standard way of getting supplies, and in doing so he created a new system of procurement, based on the hospital fund, which most large Confederate hospitals eventually emulated.

Hospitals received most of their supplies from the Quartermaster's Department, medical purveyors, and the Commissary Department through the requisition process. The necessary forms were filled out and sent to the appropriate department by the surgeons-in-charge of Chimborazo's five hospital divisions after they had learned what was needed from the stewards, matrons, and surgeons.

Upon receipt of any items, the hospital's administrators filed a report, stating the number of items received and the date on which they had arrived. If a problem arose during the process, the surgeon-in-charge appealed to McCaw, who would contact the appropriate department or, if necessary, write to Moore's office.

If the hospitals needed building materials, furniture, tents, fuel, forage, straw, non-medical equipment, clothing, stationery, or transportation, administrators sent requisitions to the Quartermaster's Department. This department, the largest supply bureau, had an extensive network of paymasters, unit quartermasters, state quartermasters, and numerous other officials assigned to specific areas. According to historian Richard Goff, some of the various duties of these officials included "purchasing forage and fuel, . . . forwarding medical stores, supervising wagon transportation in and around [Richmond], directing wagon and ambulance construction . . . supervising canal and river transportation, paying hospital accounts, and supervising state soldiers' relief associations."[2] As an independent army post, Chimborazo had its own quartermasters; this arrangement facilitated efforts to obtain supplies more quickly. Colonel A. S. Buford, Charles Werthan, and James F. West served as quartermasters at Chimborazo and ran the central office there.

Throughout the war the department routinely sent building materials and tents to Chimborazo. The quartermasters also authorized and supervised the building of the hospital's facilities; Chimborazo's carpenters did the actual construction. Several requisitions to the quartermaster list items that obviously were used to construct new wards. One such requisition, dated August 29, 1863, included requests for two thousand feet of one-inch-thick plank, five hundred pieces of three-fourths-inch plank, three thousand shingles, and various smaller pieces of strips and "scanthing."[3] Bricks, nails, cooking stoves and ward stoves, and even glass and putty were also requisitioned by McCaw for the hospital. Lime, usually ordered twenty-five barrels at a time, appears regularly in Chimborazo's requisitions to the quartermaster. The requests for these items revealed the expansion and maintenance of the hospital's buildings.[4]

To reach the hospital's maximum capacity of eight thousand patients, many patients had to be housed in tents. Both walled and Sibley tents were used. The walled tents, designed to comfortably accommodate eight patients, were 14 feet long; 14.5 feet wide; 11 feet tall in the center; and 4.5 feet tall on the outside wall. The tents could be joined end to end if desired. The entire tent was covered with a fly (21.5 by 14 feet), which could be used alone to shelter wounded "when it was inconvenient or impracticable to pitch the entire tent."[5] Conically shaped Sibley tents, 18 feet in diameter at the base and 12 feet high, were used less frequently. Surgeons mainly used these tents to isolate small numbers of highly contagious patients. Commenting on these tents, Carrington wrote, "The absence of any wall renders it inconvenient . . . for hospital purposes, and the want of a fly renders it almost intolerable on account of heat in mid-summer, while the centre pole

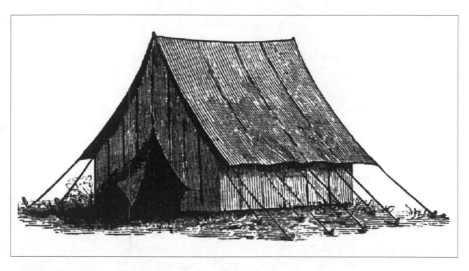

Regulation hospital tent. From *The Medical and Surgical History of the Civil War* (1870–88; reprint, Wilmington, N.C.: Broadfoot Publishing Co., 1990), vol. 12: 920.

curtails the available space and interferes with the free movements of the medical officers and attendants."[6]

Convalescent patients and patients who were only slightly wounded or sick were transferred to the tents, leaving all available beds and mattresses for those more seriously sick or wounded. In May and June of 1864, Chimborazo's census skyrocketed because of the Virginia Campaign. At that time so many tents were erected to hold the convalescents that Carrington directed McCaw to form a temporary convalescent division. On June 1, 1864, he further ordered, "If tents cannot contain them all, let them bivouac around them."[7] Major W. G. Bentley of the Quartermaster's Department wrote to McCaw on June 6, informing him, "I have just this moment come into possession of poles sufficient to set up one hundred wall tents and send them herewith with the Tents & flies."[8] By September the crisis had passed, and McCaw was instructed to return all tents, pins, and poles that his hospitals were not using.[9]

The quartermaster was also responsible for providing the hospital's bunks, benches, and tables. Chimborazo's carpenters built most of the furniture and relied only on the quartermaster to provide the materials for the bedding. The bunks of Chimborazo's patients held either mattresses or straw beds; the latter were used "in all cases which involve[d] the probability of soiling the beds."[10] In regular barracks, army regulations allowed twelve pounds of straw per soldier per month for bedding. Hospitals were not limited to a set amount; the surgeons requisitioned the amounts needed.[11]

The Quartermaster's Department also provided clothing for patients. Soldiers could receive needed clothing as soon as they became patients in the hospital. The head matron of each hospital supervised the distribution of all the clothing and bedding. All torn clothing was mended by the laundresses if possible. The head matron had to inspect all clothing considered not repairable by the laundresses. If she agreed, the material was torn to make bandages.[12] If the hospital distributed pay, clothing, or other basic supplies to patients, the surgeons-in-charge were supposed to forward duplicates of the appropriate invoices to the patients' company commanders "as soon or prior to their discharge" so that the commanders could make "duly certified returns" to their quartermaster.[13] A good idea in theory, this practice was probably followed only rarely because of the magnitude of effort

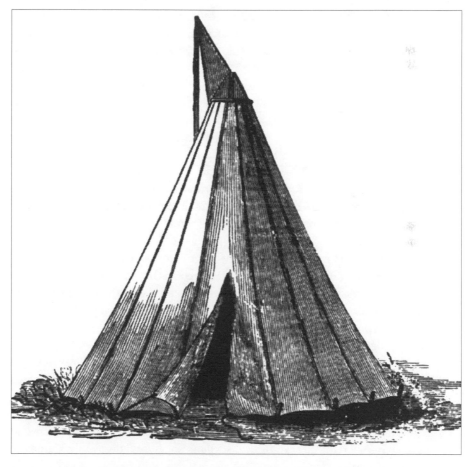

Sibley tent. From *The Medical and Surgical History of the Civil War* (1870–88; reprint, Wilmington, N.C.: Broadfoot Publishing Co., 1990), vol. 12: 920.

involved in forwarding invoices for Chimborazo's thousands of patients. The hospital's staff, including the nurses, had to provide their own clothing.[14]

Although the Quartermaster's Department did a reasonably good job of providing Chimborazo with the basic supplies, McCaw took matters into his own hands at various points during the war. One example of this involved insufficient numbers of stoves and amounts of fuel. The lack of fires concerned many of Chimborazo's staff, especially after 1863. Phoebe Pember wrote the following in her memoirs: "Stoves in any degree of newness or usefulness we did not have; they were rare and expensive luxuries. As may be supposed, they were not the most convenient articles in the world to pack away in blockade-running vessels."[15] Because of the scarcity of stoves, medical directors required surgeons-in-charge of hospitals to evaluate the situation and report how many stoves would be absolutely necessary for their institutions each winter. A report from Winder Hospital's Second Division illustrated the disbursement. Each of its twenty-two wards received two stoves each. Five stoves were placed in the kitchen, eight more were needed for food preparation in the matron's quarters, the laundry received two, and the clerks' office and dispensary received one each.[16]

McCaw worked hard to find an adequate number of stoves for his hospital, but when that had been accomplished, obtaining the fuel to fire the stoves was another challenge. Keeping the wards properly heated in the winter was a problem throughout the war, especially with the harshness of the winters during those years. In the 1862–63 winter, Richmond recorded twenty-seven snowfalls.[17] Even at the beginning of the war, the surgeon general wrote to McCaw of "the great difficulty of furnishing fuel."[18] To remedy this situation, McCaw furnished the wood for his hospitals for the first two years of Chimborazo's operation, "during which time there was an ample supply." However, the "quartermaster declined to permit this arrangement to continue," which resulted in the hospital being "inadequately supplied."[19] In November and December of 1863, Chimborazo No. 4 had fifty-one stoves but averaged only twenty-six fires: eighteen in the wards, five for cooking, and one each in the surgeons' office, the steward's office, and the druggists' office. The Surgeon General's Office asked McCaw for a detailed report regarding the current amount and type of fuel consumed, the number and placement of fires, and the number of fires needed if the hospital's wards became filled with patients. When McCaw responded with the information, he requested 240 cords of wood and 75 bushels of coal for 130 fires for his twelve hundred patients and attendants for the month of February.[20] The quality of the fuel lessened as the war continued. By 1864 Pember explained, "[T]he trouble and expense of land transportation also seriously affected the quality of wood for fuel, furnished us. Timber which had been condemned heretofore as unfit for use, light, soggy, and decayed, became the only quality available."[21]

From Chimborazo's records, it appears that all fuel requisitions from the hospital were granted until the winter of 1864, when some orders were reduced. For the month of October 1864, McCaw requested 150 cords of wood to heat the fires for two thousand patients and attendants; he received only 100 cords. For January 1865, he only received 200 of the 300 cords requested.[22] Throughout that winter the reports of the officer of the day at Chimborazo No. 2 continually lamented the lack of wood. On November 3, 1864, medical officer John Jackson wrote, "Convalescent patients had taken their beds to keep warm."[23]

Another example of McCaw's devotion to providing for the hospital concerned the adequate and timely payment of his staff. Payment of the wages of the hospital's staff and patients was the responsibility of the Quartermaster's Department, which also provided the funds for the commutation of quarters and fuel for its surgeons.[24] Evidently, the department sometimes postponed payment of wages when funds were tight. One source stated, "The hospitals have . . . been embarrassed by the non-payment of the hospital attendants by the Quartermaster's Department."[25] McCaw attempted to alleviate any hardship caused by a lack of wages by using the hospital fund in whatever ways he could. McCaw also worked to obtain the best employees by paying his workers as much as possible. When he attempted to pay his stewards more than regulations allowed, he was rebuked by Surgeon General Moore, especially since he had taken the amount from the hospital fund.[26] He also used the fund to pay for the rooms in Richmond that the matrons rented, although Moore disapproved of that practice as well.[27]

Another group McCaw worked with and around consisted of the medical purveyors, all of whom were surgeons or assistant surgeons, appointed by the surgeon general. Medical purveyors handled almost all of the money appropriated to the Medical Department by the Confederate government. They worked under the authority of the surgeon general to procure and distribute goods designated as medical and hospital supplies to the military hospitals in their region. By November 1864 there were thirty-two medical purveyors in the Confederacy. Surgeon Edward W. Johns served as the medical purveyor assigned to Richmond. From the beginning of the war through mid-1864, Edward Johns received fifty-four warrants from the Treasury Department, totaling $4,143,478.58 for medical supplies in the Richmond area.[28]

Although it would seem that medical purveyors had a great deal of money at their disposal, they had to provide a variety of articles. In addition to medications, alcohol, medical instruments, and medical textbooks, purveyors also had to provide goods considered important to the care of the Confederacy's patients. The following items from the supply table illustrate the diversity: bed sacks, coverlets, pillow ticks, sheets, mosquito bars, bandages, corks, red flannel, lint, medicine cups and glasses, coffee mills, muslin, sewing needles, bed pans, paper envelopes, wrapping paper, writing paper, pencils, rain gauges, razors, tape, towels, urinals, and assorted vials. Items such as wash basins, bowls, buckets, candlesticks, tea kettles, forks, spoons, mugs, lanterns, pitchers, coffee pots, chamber pots, tumblers, and woodsaws could be procured from the medical purveyor or quartermaster by special requisition.[29] Medical purveyors also provided hospitals with medical textbooks on a variety of subjects. According to the supply table, each hospital was allowed one copy of a book on each of the following subjects: anatomy, chemistry, dispensing medications, medical jurisprudence and toxicology, medical practice, obstetrics, and surgery. A medical dictionary and two copies of the Medical Department's regulations were also allowed for each hospital.

Because of the great demand for supplies and the corresponding possibility of corruption, the purveyors and quartermasters both implemented an invoicing system to track supplies. The invoice was enclosed with any goods sent to the hospital. When the packages arrived at Chimborazo, the hospital's staff helped the teamsters unload the supplies. The medical officers then inspected the packages so that they could report back to the medical purveyor about when the supplies arrived, the number of packages received, and whether they corresponded with the invoice.[30] At times, the medical officers had to be reminded of their duty to send the receipt invoice. On December 7, 1863, the Quartermaster's Department wrote to McCaw asking for the third time for verification of some potatoes sent to Chimborazo.[31] The next month, the Surgeon General's Office also complained, reminding McCaw that Medical Department regulations required the receipts: "No returns of medical supplies which came into your hands while in charge of Chimborazo Hospl have been received at this office for the 1/2 year ending 30 June 1863."[32]

If the supplies arrived in a damaged or unusable condition, a report on their condition had to be made. If the receiving persons failed to make a report, they could later be held responsible for any shortages. In 1864 McCaw ordered a board of survey formed of medical officers to "examine & report upon an invoice of Shoes." A box of shoes, invoiced as containing a hundred pairs, was found to contain only ninety-four pairs. After investigating, the board reported that the box "upon being opened was apparently full. . . . We do exonerate Capt West from all blame or responsibility because of the loss of said shoes."[33] Evidently, this board of survey continued to investigate supply discrepancies. When some damaged socks arrived at Chimborazo, the board reported that the socks were "in a damaged condition when received by Capt Jas. F. West AQM." It exonerated him from all blame, then recommended "that he issue the said damaged socks to servants."[34]

Hospital and medical supplies were especially hard to obtain, as the Union army early in the war had declared medications and surgical instruments to be contraband. Thus, most Confederate medical supplies had to be either smuggled into the South through the blockade or manufactured by the Confederacy. Providing medications was the most obvious problem. To meet the challenge, Moore took three major steps. First, he prohibited the sale of critical medications to anyone other than government purchasing officers.[35] Second, he ordered pharmaceutical laboratories established in Atlanta and Macon, Georgia; Columbia and Charleston, South Carolina; Charlotte and Lincolnton, North Carolina; Montgomery and Mobile, Alabama; and Tyler, Texas. Later in the war other labs were opened. Medical purveyors controlled the laboratories, employing pharmacists and chemists to analyze and produce medicines. Some of the medications were copies of existing drugs; others were substitutes made from native roots and herbs. Some substitutes, such as wild jalep for ipecac, were successful; others, such as jasmine or wild cherry for foxglove, were of little value. "Indigenous and other products manufactured at the depots were also examined closely; hence the laboratories served both as manufacturing laboratories and as analytical control stations."[36]

When the Confederate laboratories discovered that opium made from the red garden poppy was just as effective as what was received from Northern pharmaceutical companies, the surgeon general instructed medical purveyors to encourage the ladies of the South "to interest themselves in the culture of the Garden Poppy." Moore continued, "Purveyors will furnish the ladies with the seeds of the Poppy if on hand or procurable, and will instruct them, that the juice exceeding from the punctured capsules, when sufficiently hardened, should be carefully put up, and forwarded to the nearest Purveying depot."[37] Many individuals and relief societies began trying to grow red poppies to meet the large demand.

As a third measure Moore encouraged his physicians to use remedies made from indigenous plant materials. His office provided information about native remedies through a pamphlet released in 1862 and a book by F. Peyre Porcher published in 1863. When Moore placed native remedies on the medical supply table in March 1863, he encouraged his officers to keep an open mind and "give them a fair opportunity for the exhibition of those remedial virtues which they certainly possess."[38] An additional benefit of using indigenous remedies was that hospitals would not have to rely on the Purveyor's Office to obtain their supply. Instead, surgeons were expected to send their attendants and convalescent patients into the neighboring countryside to gather the plants when needed.[39]

Even though shortages of medical supplies have received much attention, the Medical Department was able to provide essential medications to its hospitals and surgeons until the very end of the war. Most of the reported shortages occurred at the very beginning of the war before the supply system was in place, or else they occurred at field hospitals far from established supply lines. The general hospitals held an advantage over those in the field. Shortages of some key medical items did threaten various regions of the Confederacy during the war, but such shortages were usually resolved within a short time.[40]

Some of the shortages lay beyond the control of the Purveyor's Office. Once the purveyor obtained the necessary supplies, he sent them to the quartermaster's depot for transportation to the hospital. Any transportation problems experienced could result in temporary shortages. In *Doctors in Gray*, H. H. Cunningham stated, "The entire complex problem of procurement and supply was complicated many times over late in the war when the Confederacy's transportation system collapsed. Wagon as well as railroad transportation broke down almost completely, and needed supplies arrived tardily at their destination, if at all."[41]

Other shortages occurred when the laboratories' production of medication increased faster than vials and boxes could be obtained. Consequently, medications could not be sent from the labs to the hospitals. To solve this problem, the medical purveyor requested that medical officers return any empty medicine vials and usable boxes when reordering supplies.[42] Moore directed Carrington to "instruct Surgeons attending Officers & soldiers sick in Private Quarters to direct that all vials, and vial corks be returned to the C.S. Dispensary as soon as the patient is done using the same."[43]

One of the items in short supply toward the end of the war was alcohol. Believed then to be a stimulant, liquor was a medication of choice for many ailments. Even in 1861 newspapers reported how the high demand of whiskey was making Confederate distillers rich. The Charleston *Mercury* reported, "the demand for whiskey was such that every gallon was sold as soon as it was made."[44] In Georgia, the state legislature found it necessary to fix the price of the precious commodity at $1.50 per gallon. Chimborazo was not hurt as much as the other hospitals from this shortage since it had a brewery that could produce as many as four hundred kegs of beer in one batch. Franklin Stearns's nearby distillery supplemented the hospital's supply. Stearns reportedly made a tremendous amount of money from this distillery during the war. In 1862 the Confederate Congress placed the distribution of this critical medicinal product for hospitals under the supervision of its head matrons in order to stop any abuses of the substance. Although this measure helped, by 1864 liquor remained in very short supply; Confederate distillers simply could not keep up with the high demand.[45]

At that point, the Medical Department took further precautions to ensure the liquor was being used properly. In July 1864, medical officers in all Confederate hospitals were instructed that all alcoholic stimulants were to be requisitioned on a form separate from the one requesting other medical and hospital supplies. The purveyor would send the alcohol "by a perfectly reliable man," who would deliver it to the hospital's surgeon-in-charge, who in turn would give it to the matron. Officers were ordered to report any "abuses or improper use" to the Surgeon General's Office.[46] In November 1864 the Surgeon General's Office issued a circular in response to the "frequent reports which reach this office relative to the abuse practiced by medical officers in the administration of alcoholic stimulants to patients and others for trivial complaints." Medical officers were informed that the "difficulty of procuring a future supply has now become a matter of deep concern," and officers were "forbidden" to prescribe alcohol "except in such cases as imperatively demand [its] administration."[47]

As the war continued, shortages of items other than medications and liquor occurred. If a surgeon needed a new set of surgical instruments, the best way to obtain one was to capture it from the enemy—a difficult feat for a hospital surgeon. If the surgeon relied on his medical purveyor, the instruments he received would most likely have been manufactured in the Confederacy. According to Lafayette Guild, medical director of the Army of Northern Virginia, those who had instruments made in the Confederacy "might as well be without any, for those they have are entirely useless."[48] Toward the end of the war, the shortage grew worse. Surgeon Johns failed to obtain any surgical instruments for issue in the Richmond area in 1864 or 1865.[49] To assist surgeons' efforts to find working instruments, an 1864 circular informed medical officers that if they sent their broken surgical instruments to Surgeon Thomas Lining, the medical purveyor in Charleston, the instruments would be "put in good order" by a man whom Lining had detailed for that special purpose.[50] Fortunately, however desperate the need for surgical equipment was in other places, Chimborazo Hospital seemed to be adequately supplied. When the hospital closed at the end of the war, thirteen cases of surgical instruments were found at the facility.[51]

The growing shortage of medical and hospital supplies in the Richmond area was illustrated by a suspicious fire that destroyed seven wards at Winder No. 2 on January 21, 1864. After orders were received to consolidate Winder's second division with its first and third, the excess inventory was stored in one of the wards of No. 2 "for safekeeping." Reportedly, this fire could not have been accidental. Two of the best attendants stated, "[T]he fire in the stove, in the middle of the building, had entirely gave out [sic]." After the fire the only items found to be intact and reusable were the windows' hinges and nails.[52]

Because of the difficulty in obtaining some supplies, hospitals such as Chimborazo recycled as much as they could. Comforters, for example, were used over and over again. Once the padding in them had been soiled and required cleaning, they were ripped open so that the infected padding could be removed. Then, either the padding was replaced, or the light cloth remaining was made into light blankets for use in the warmer seasons.[53] When the cloth became too bare for use as blankets, attendants tore it into strips to use as bandages. When the padding and feathers became harder to obtain, the hospitals commonly used corn offal and other substitutes. By the last months of the war, surgeons and their staffs became creative in finding ways to stuff their patients' mattresses. Carrington informed McCaw of this situation:

> I fear that neither straw, shucks or any other article that can be used as
> long forage can be procured to fill beds at the Hospl. [sic] You are

directed to examine into the Merits of any and all suitable substitutes that suggest themselves to you as readily procurable and report to this office. The smaller rags, tufts, or tops, of pine trees, oak leaves, or shavings or sawdust from Carpenter Shops occur to me.[54]

Not only hospitals recycled materials. Starting in 1863, the surgeon general encouraged medical purveyors to collect all surplus scraps "remaining from the manufacture of Hospital clothing, and to dispose of the same to the nearest paper manufacturers, either for cash, or in exchange for paper."[55]

The Commissary Department was responsible for providing food to all Confederate soldiers, including those in the hospital. However, only very rarely did the department send any food to Chimborazo or other similar hospitals.[56] The sick and wounded required a nutritious and varied diet to regain their strength. Frequently, the commissary could not easily obtain perishable items such as vegetables, fruit, eggs, and milk. Even when it could, the department's policy to issue the stores longest on hand often resulted in perishables that were unfit for use. Recognizing the ineffectiveness of its efforts to provide perishable goods, the commissary usually sent only non-perishable goods to the hospitals and sent the remainder of the funds from the patients' rations to a hospital fund, which the hospital's administrator could use at his discretion to purchase perishable and other "luxury" items for his patients. The commuted value of a soldier's daily ration began at $.75; then increased to $1.00 on September 27, 1862; then to $1.25 on May 1, 1863; and finally to $2.50 on February 25, 1864.[57] At the beginning of the war, the ration of a hospital patient was more than that of a soldier. However, as the war continued and shortages grew, the hospital ration decreased until it became the same for all soldiers, sick or healthy, in December 1863.[58]

All military hospitals, Union and Confederate, had a hospital fund, but McCaw made particularly creative use of his. Instead of being forced to spend most of the money in his hospital fund on food, McCaw built his institution to produce much of what his hospital needed. He set aside some of the hospital's leased acreage, which became known as the farm, to graze milk cows and raise other livestock for hospital use. He also ordered the planting of a large vegetable garden and used the hospital fund for the necessary seed and equipment for the garden. Convalescent patients and detailed men provided the labor, and the stables provided the manure.

Evidently, Surgeon General Moore was convinced of the wisdom of hospital gardens by 1864. In February of that year, he ordered the medical directors of hospitals to "call attention . . . to the importance of immediate steps being taken by them to provide an abundant supply of vegetables for their Hospital for the present year" and declared, "Hospital gardens should be established without delay."[59] By this point army hospital administrators could obtain seeds for their gardens from the Commissary Department. Hospital gardens were used successfully throughout the Confederacy, except in the hospitals that were forced to remain mobile.[60]

Chimborazo's bakery provided most of the bread for the hospital's patients and staff, except for black attendants, who were not allowed to have bread made from flour. At its peak operation, the bakery could produce ten thousand loaves of bread per day. The matrons' kitchens made the bread for the very sick patients. Bread was a major staple in the diet at the hospital. Each patient and white attendant received one pound of bread by weight per day.[61] The bakery obtained its flour from the Commissary Department. One pound of flour or one pound of potatoes resulted in one pound nine ounces of bread. At Chimborazo, Hospital No. 3 provided the grease for the pans at the bakery.

According to Medical Department regulations, all other expenses of the bakery, including the wages of the baker and his five hired hands, came from the hospital fund. When Chimborazo first opened, McCaw detailed Private William Bowers as the baker.[62] For most of the war, however, George Gates managed the bakery at Chimborazo. In addition to Gates, seven other men worked in the bakery. His major helper was paid fourteen dollars per week plus board. Of the rest of the staff, four hands were black, and two were "hirelings . . . , and the 2 put in one would hardly make a man." Gates used between one and one-and-a-half pounds of hops and one-and-a-half cords of wood per week. In a letter to McCaw, Gates stated, "I want to work as economical and deep of expenses of you as much as as [*sic*] I can." Gates illustrated his thriftiness by pointing out that although "every Baker in Richmond uses malt," he did not use malt for his bread since it would come to nine dollars more per month.[63]

By 1864 shortages affected even bread production. In January McCaw informed the surgeons-in-charge, "[T]he Bakery is discontinued owing to want of flour. Corn meal will be furnished for the Genl Kitchens & attendants in suitable quantities. Flour will be issued to the Matrons at the rate of 33 1/3 pounds for 100 men."[64] Of that summer Pember wrote, "[E]very ounce of flour was valuable. . . . After the flour or meal had been made into bread, it was almost ludicrous to see with what painful solicitude Miss G. and myself would count the rolls, or hold a council over pans of corn-bread, measuring with a string how large we could afford to cut the squares."[65] Although the closing of the bakery was temporary, it dramatically illustrated the shortages experienced in even the most basic of supplies. When it reopened, production of bread was cut because of the continued shortage of wheat and other necessary ingredients. Chimborazo No. 1 drew approximately 160 pounds of bread per day from the bakery in late October 1864.[66] Chimborazo No. 3 received 1,890 pounds of bread for its patients from December 21 to December 31, 1864. The bakery had used 1,496 pounds of flour to make that amount of bread. The amount of bread distributed to the other four hospitals at Chimborazo was similar. Because this statistic was from late in the war, many shortages had decreased the amount of bread distributed. The shortages had also closed most of the bakeries in Richmond.[67]

Another way in which Chimborazo provided for itself was through the manufacture of much of its own soap. At Chimborazo, a "Mr. Miles" ran the soaphouse. He used the leftover grease from the kitchens of Chimborazo Nos. 1, 2, 4, and 5. From June 13 to October 20, 1864, Chimborazo No. 5 alone furnished Miles with 543 pounds of grease and drew approximately 1,350 pounds of soap from him.[68] By the end of the war, the ashes of wheat straw were also used to make soap. When the straw mattresses on patients' beds became unfit for use, the straw was burned to provide the necessary ashes. This practice assured that the foul straw was disposed of properly and also saved funds that would have been spent on soap.[69]

Unfortunately, not all of Chimborazo's requirements could be met by on-site production. When obtaining food supplies from the hospital's garden and the Purveyor's Office failed, the hospital relied upon the talents of its hospital agents for food. I. I. Lindsey and Thomas W. Scott, among others, served as the supply agents for Chimborazo Hospital. The price of food in Richmond and other cities was outrageous because of the high demand from its overcrowded population. As the population of Richmond exploded in 1861 and 1862, the demand for food raised prices dramatically. By January 1863, food costs in Richmond were ten times what they had been in 1860.[70] To combat the rising local prices, the hospital agents traveled throughout the surrounding countryside to procure vegetables, eggs, and meat for their hospitals through purchases from farmers and gardeners.

Once a connection had been made between Chimborazo and a farmer, usually more than one transaction followed. Charles W. Arnold, a farmer from Petersburg, wrote to McCaw on January 20, 1863, offering to sell 150 bushels of peas "at the same price of the last lot sold to Mr. Tho. W. Scott for your Hospital." A letter was sent the next day, accepting the price of five dollars per bushel; the peas were shipped on January 23.[71]

Other hospitals soon followed Chimborazo's example, and competition developed between agents from different hospitals. On August 13, 1863, McCaw and the other surgeons-in-charge of hospitals in the Richmond area met, as ordered by Carrington, "to arrange some common schedule of prices for articles bought with the Hospital Fund." This action was necessary because the Medical Department had discovered that "in the expenditure of the Hospital Fund competition and want of cooperation [had] enhanced prices to the injury of the Government and the encouragement of extortion."[72] By the end of the war, the Surgeon General's Office warned agents that they were carefully watching the prices paid for hospital supplies; "the Surgeon in charge [would] be held strictly responsible for any extravagance in price."[73]

Once a purchase was made, transporting the goods to the hospital became the challenge, especially when dealing with perishable items. In a December 1862 note to McCaw, supply agent Thomas Scott informed McCaw that he had obtained pota-toes, soap, and butter for the hospital but had been unable to find a way to trans-port them to Chimborazo.[74] Transportation of items was problematic in the early years of the war. To remedy the situation, McCaw used the hospital fund to pur-chase wagons that the agents could use.

Another advantage Chimborazo had with regard to transportation was the trading canal boat, named the *Chimborazo*. Lawrence Lottier commanded the boat "which traded between Richmond and Lexington, [on the Kanawa Canal] barter-ing cotton yarns, shoes, newbys, etc., for provisions."[75] Surprisingly, only Chim-borazo and its sister hospital Winder had boats to transport supplies.[76] The canal boats gave the hospital's agents an extended reach to find food and supplies and a way to transport items more quickly than over land. This advantage grew as competition for items in the Richmond area became extreme. Chimborazo's agents were able to keep their expenses down by extending their search beyond the sur-rounding countryside. Much correspondence survives between Chimborazo's agents and McCaw; some letters were sent from as far away as North Carolina.

As food and other supplies became increasingly difficult to find, commission merchant companies, such as Kent, Paine, and Kent, helped the hospital's agents to locate food and supplies. News of available miscellaneous supplies was sometimes discovered through Carrington as well. In October 1864 Carrington informed McCaw about a man in Halifax County who was making brooms to sell at four dol-lars each. "They are said to be very superior," Carrington wrote. "Will you want any at that price?"[77]

The price problem was exacerbated as the value of Confederate currency declined. By mid-January 1865, one Union dollar was worth seventy Confederate dollars; by the end of February, its worth had fallen further—to one hundred Confederate dollars for each Union greenback.[78] In the later years of the war, many citizens with food to sell refused to be paid with Confederate money, preferring instead to trade their food for goods the hospitals had. For the hospitals he over-saw in the Army of Tennessee, Samuel Stout "authorized trading brown earthen ware pottery, made specifically for the hospitals, for food supplies," according to his biographer, Glenna Schroeder-Lein.[79]

In 1864 and 1865, Chimborazo's self-sufficiency and agents' networks became more important as the food available in the Richmond area grew more scarce. However, even with its advantages, the large hospital could not obtain a sufficient amount of food. Surgeon Tobias G. Richardson wrote of this shortage in March 1864 after touring Chimborazo, Winder, and Jackson Hospitals. Comparing those hospitals to the ones in the Army of Tennessee, Richardson informed Stout, "[I]n feeding [your hospitals] are infinitely superior. Indeed it is almost impossible for any one to get enough to eat, either outside or inside the hospitals, for the simple reason that it is not to be had at any price."[80]

When shortages of various items became serious, McCaw increased security at Chimborazo. On October 1, 1863, he instructed Chimborazo's guard "to arrest any one going out of the Hospl with Bread or any other provisions & keep them in the Guard House until he reports . . . to me."[81] Two days later McCaw released a notice: "No Provisions or Hospital Property of any sort are to be sent past the guard unless with an order from Capt. Ferrell . . . or with a certificate from the Surg in Chg of Division that they are intended for the use of a patient. The guard is to be rigid in making arrests."[82]

In addition to increased security, some rationing occurred. In December 1863 Moore released a circular directing hospitals not to use coffee anymore as part of their patients' diets. He explained, "In consequence of the very limited supply, it is essential that it be used soley [*sic*] for its medicinal effects as a stimulant."[83]

At the same time, ironically, the supply of other items seemed to be abundant. Carrington released a circular in October 1863, instructing the surgeons-in-charge of general hospitals "to receive *all* sweet potatoes turned over to them." The circular then provided instructions on how to winter the potatoes.[84] Later that same month, steward H. B. Gaines wrote to McCaw, asking if he should buy the fourteen or sixteen bushels of sweet potatoes that Mrs. W. & G. Gwathmey offered him at market rates.[85]

Throughout the war McCaw used the money in Chimborazo's hospital fund to its best advantage. Although he worked through the appropriate channels when possible, he determinedly refused to let policy and tradition keep him from acting in what he knew to be the best interests of his hospital. Chimborazo's records reveal several instances when the surgeon general rebuked McCaw for not following the correct procedure to obtain supplies. In a letter on February 18, 1863, Moore chastised McCaw for purchasing wagons, a horse, and liquors directly, instead of going through the medical purveyor. Moore explained that if the amount allowed by the supply table "were found insufficient," McCaw must still go through official channels.[86]

The month before, McCaw had purchased bacon with money from the hospital fund. Moore refused to honor the voucher sent to his office by McCaw, returning it with a note of explanation to Chimborazo's administrator:

> If the Bacon obtained from the Commissary is unsuited for the use
> of the sick in Hospital or is insufficient in quantity, a proper report of
> such facts should be made by you to this office that measures may be
> taken for the correction of the cause of complaint, but the [hospital]
> fund must not be used for the almost entire provisioning of the
> Hospital when supplies can be obtained from the government by
> requisition.[87]

However, the Medical Department's approach softened as the medical purveyor's department began to have difficulty obtaining a sufficient amount of goods. In December 1863 Moore authorized officers to purchase blank books and stationery as needed—after checking with the purveyor to make sure he did not have any available, of course.[88] By this point, McCaw's use of the fund had gone much beyond buying paper, and Carrington evidently approved of his liberal use of the fund. In mid-1864 Carrington wrote to McCaw suggesting that he "draw the necessary hospital funds . . . to enable [him] to buy mules or horses sufficient to supply an additional ambulance for each Division of the Hospital under your charge."[89] By the end of the war, the only way McCaw could not use the hospital fund was to purchase medicines, which was prohibited by law except for the purveyors.

Another means that McCaw used to purchase necessary items was by the development of a "post fund," for which Chimborazo, as an independent army post, qualified. Any bread produced in Chimborazo's bakery that was not eaten by the patients was allowed to be sold to the public. Beginning in March 1863, as a result of a proposal by McCaw to Moore, the profits from the bakery became designated as the post fund.[90] Separate from the hospital fund, this fund was similar to a modern-day petty-cash fund and allowed McCaw even more flexibility in determining how to pay for items he considered essential.

Even with its liberal use, Chimborazo's hospital fund consistently remained in the black. The excess in the fund relieved the hospital of one problem that its sister institutions faced. Evidently, at various points in the war the Commissary Department was delinquent in depositing the commuted rations into the hospital's fund.[91] In an interview after the war, McCaw stated, "[A]t the close of the war the Confederate Government owed us three hundred thousand dollars."[92] McCaw seemed to be proud of Chimborazo's self-sufficiency: "We never drew fifty dollars from the Confederate States Government, but relied solely upon the money received from commutation of our rations."[93]

Chimborazo also periodically received food and supplies from state contributions and donations from charitable groups and individuals. At various points in the war, and especially after the hospitals were designated to serve patients from a particular home state, individual states donated money and supplies for the use of their soldiers who were patients in the hospital. In 1864 Carrington informed McCaw that several congressmen from Tennessee would be visiting Chimborazo No. 4, which housed all patients from that state. The congressmen wanted to provide money "to expend for the comfort of their fellow statesmen."[94] Later that same year, O. F. Manson, medical agent of the state of North Carolina, wrote to McCaw to request a list—arranged by name, rank, and regiment—of all sick and wounded patients from North Carolina. Manson stated, "Should their necessities require anything in the line of Medicines clothing or food, which cannot be obtained in sufficient quantity, please make a requisition & I will forward it to the governor of NC."[95] An admirable gesture, this requisition process probably took much too long to be practical.

Charitable groups in the North similarly played a critical role in keeping Union troops and patients well supplied. The United States Sanitary Commission organized over seven thousand aid societies, which sent supplies to their local USSC chapter. Those chapters in turn sent them to one of ten regional warehouses and then on to one of two central depots. Hired USSC agents distributed the donated supplies as soon as they received a request or anticipated a shortage.[96] The charitable groups in the South did not have the organization or effectiveness of their Northern counterparts but still contributed a great deal to the war effort.

Soon after the war began, charity societies were formed throughout the South to help provide food, clothing, and other necessary items to the soldiers. Although Chimborazo and other hospitals did not rely on the charitable contributions, all materials provided by charities were, of course, greatly appreciated and encouraged. In Chimborazo's files, the following announcement illustrated the eagerness of the hospital to receive charitable goods.

> A depot for the Virginia troops having been established by the
> state on Shockoe Slip Richmond near Columbian Hotel the people
> will have the opportunity of doing much for the comfort of the sick
> & wounded & all contributions of clothing, books, & comforts of
> every description will be thankfully received and duly forwarded
> by Mr. A. S. Buford, State Agent.[97]

Phoebe Pember explained the importance of the goods sent from the various charitable associations and from individual state governments. "[I]mmense contributions, coming weekly from these sources, gave great aid, and enabled [the hospital] to have a reserve store when government supplies failed," she recalled.[98]

A list of some of the items sent to Chimborazo by the Ladies Cumberland Hospital Association illustrates the extensive quantity and variety of charitable donations. Besides cash, the LCHA sent basic items such as shirts, drawers, pants, socks, cotton and linen bandages, pillow cases, lint, and soap. Food items donated included one hundred chickens, hams, eggs, butter, honey, onions, sweet potatoes, apples, blackberries, pickles, catsup, bread, and cakes. The association also sent brandy and wine, as well as miscellaneous items such as fans.[99]

In Richmond, the Ladies Aid Society, led by Mrs. George Randolph, was the major charity organization. Throughout the war the society gave a great deal to help the Confederate cause. However, the diarist Mary Chesnut revealed some of the problems that limited its effectiveness, many of which might have been avoided if a national, or even regional, leadership structure had been in place. In the early months of the war, when Richmond was completely overrun with wounded in its various makeshift hospitals, the Ladies Aid Society focused on contributing to the hospitals. Soon, however, the desperate need for supplies in all parts of the Confederate army caused the group to shift its attention to the most recently revealed shortage, and the hospitals were left to fend for themselves. Throughout her diary Chesnut reported one "small war" in the society after another, caused by disagreements about which group was most deserving or which need was most pressing. One of the first controversies centered on whether the group would contribute any aid to the captured Yankee wounded who were in Confederate hospitals.[100]

Another problem was the waning enthusiasm of some Ladies Aid Society members as the war continued past its first months. On September 19, 1861, Chesnut wrote, "At first there were nearly a hundred members—eighty or ninety always present at a meeting—now ten or twenty are all that they can show. The worse is, they have forgotten the hospitals, where they really could do so much good, and gone off to provision and clothe the army. A drop in the bucket—or ocean."[101] Chesnut's entry for October 15, 1861, revealed another aspect of the waning enthusiasm on the part of Richmond's women. "Shocked to hear," she wrote, "that dear friends of mine refused to take work for the soldiers because their sempstresses [sic] had their winter clothes to make. I told them true patriotesses would be willing to wear the same clothes until our siege was raised."[102]

The Southern tendency to give charitably to soldiers from one's home state also limited the effectiveness of the charities. In the August 5, 1861, entry in her journal, Chesnut reported that she had been rebuked that day by Sally Tompkins because she had asked if there were any Carolinians in Miss Tompkins's hospital. Tompkins reportedly replied, "I never ask where the sick and wounded come from." Although Chesnut conceded that the rebuke was deserved, she wrote on August 23 that she had given provisions to "our Carolinians" at Tompkins's hospital.[103]

Success in the supplies realm greatly contributed to more contented patients and staff and to a more effective hospital. The lack of general supplies not only caused discomfort for the patients but also hindered the number of patients that Chimborazo could receive for treatment. For example, the morning report of Chimborazo Hospital No. 4 on July 17, 1862, reported how the lack of straw, used to stuff patients' mattresses, could prevent new patients from being received: "By reason of a large number of wounded the demand for clean bed sacks is heavy— There are 100 vacant beds but not so many clean beds ready for them." A month later, the situation had scarcely improved. The surgeon stated, "For want of straw patients cannot be received to full capacity of hosp [sic]."[104]

Even though the supplies situation at Chimborazo Hospital was less than perfect, the self-sufficiency of Chimborazo helped provide basic food and limited the hospital's reliance on outside sources. Its size, network of agents, and means of transportation allowed the hospital to bring goods in from a distance. Its reputation helped Chimborazo's agents to purchase goods when others failed. Towards the end of the war, Chimborazo did experience shortages of various items, but those items were not available to anyone in the region. At the very end of the war, when the hospital closed, Pember reported its commissary full.[105] Very few hospitals or camps could make similar claims.

Considering the size of Chimborazo and the enormity of the supplies challenge, the success of the hospital's staff in this area is notable. If McCaw had failed in this single area, then his hospital would have been viewed and remembered negatively; the lack of supplies would have overshadowed all its accomplishments. Instead, the ingenuity of McCaw and his talented agents helped ensure that Chimborazo was as well supplied as possible. Through his liberal use of the hospital fund, guided by the concept of improving overall patient care, McCaw showed how well he understood the importance of solving the basic physical problems of his hospital as well as the medical problems of his patients. The lack of frustration about the supplies issue allowed the medical staff to do their jobs to the best of their abilities without being hindered by shortages of food or other critical items. Because the hospital could obtain supplies, its patients and staff could focus their attention on the other aspects of life at Chimborazo.

CHAPTER 6

Medical Treatment

Most studies of the medical treatment received by Confederate and Union soldiers during the Civil War elicit shock and disbelief from readers. From a twenty-first century perspective, many of the beliefs about the causes of disease and the treatments for disease seem ignorant at best and barbaric at worst. Works on Civil War medicine usually begin with some statistics on how many men died during the conflict and that "two soldiers died of diseases for every one killed in battle."[1] Often these numbers prompt a negative assumption about the medical treatment during the war. Most of the details provided encourage this assumption by focusing on incompetent or uncaring surgeons or on the periods of extreme medical crisis, such as occurred after the battles at Antietam or Gettysburg. For these reasons, according to Peter J. Parish, "numerous historians have concluded that 'the medical services represent one of the Civil War's most dismal failures.'"[2] An obvious target on which to pin the blame for this "failure" is the corps of physicians who supervised the medical treatment. However, as discussed in previous chapters, the competence of physicians was guaranteed, on at least a minimum level, by examinations before army boards composed of experienced surgeons. Most physicians were not the ignorant, incompetent buffoons portrayed by past literature but were in fact thoughtful medical professionals, doing the best they could with the existing medical knowledge of the time. So, what does explain the problem? Keeping in mind the medical knowledge and standards of the time, no problem existed.

As we examine the different medical treatments common at Chimborazo and other large Civil War hospitals, the reasons for their medical success and relatively low mortality rates will give balance to the medical horror stories of the same period. Although the numbers are striking and horror stories abound, the real story of Civil War medical treatment should focus on how many sick and wounded patients survived. The two-to-one ratio of deaths from disease to battle deaths comes into perspective when measured against other nineteenth-century military conflicts: eight to one in the Napoleonic Wars, seven to one in the Mexican War (1846–48), almost four to one in Britain's Crimean War (1854–56), and six to one in the Spanish-American War (1898).[3]

In many ways, the best viewpoint from which to examine medical treatment during the war is the setting of the general hospital. Since field hospitals generally transported their critical patients and their long-term convalescents to the general hospitals, extended treatment in the mobile facilities was uncommon. The lack of extended treatment and the instability of the physical situation of the field hospitals prohibited surgeons from keeping clinical records on patients. Also, the mortality rates of field hospitals were skewed by the number of critically wounded patients beyond medical help; any statistics would also be unreliable because of the high numbers of patients transferred to general hospitals. The mobility of field hospitals presented their medical staffs with challenges that focused their attention on keeping patients alive, which hindered their capacity to stay on the cutting edge of medical knowledge and treatments. Finding an adequate site to set up their hospital to deal with the wounded after a battle and operating on hundreds of patients in a high-stress environment were the main concerns of the field surgeons.

Because of the permanent nature of general hospitals, the medical treatment there could be better conceived and more deliberate. The lower chance of being transferred out of the general hospital increased the consistency of medical treatment. One or two physicians became familiar with the patients in their wards and knew their medical histories. Also, the larger general hospitals enabled the physicians to see many patients who had the same illness, or at least similar symptoms. Patterns became familiar to the doctors, who then worked to find treatments that could help their patients recover. Through the hierarchy of medical officers at a general hospital, the knowledge and supervision of the more experienced surgeons helped to offset any inexperience the assistant surgeons or contract surgeons might have. The large pool of medical officers at a hospital allowed for a debate and exchange of ideas when a particularly difficult case developed.

The medical treatment received by patients at Chimborazo Hospital was as good or better than at any other hospital during the Civil War. A look at the medical treatment at Chimborazo or any other Civil War hospital does not reveal huge medical advances. However, if one examines the medical records closely, an understanding of the clinical, scientific nature of medical practice in this era becomes obvious, especially at Chimborazo. The intellectual environment at Chimborazo Hospital, fostered by Dr. McCaw, encouraged debate and open-mindedness on medical issues and provided the stable administrative situation to support the advancement of medical knowledge.

Chimborazo Hospital had many advantages over other general hospitals. First of all, not only did its location remain the same throughout the war, but it was also built to be a hospital. Its one-story pavilion design—a progressive feature—allowed for a more healthy environment than multistoried buildings. An abundance of clean water from nearby springs and a varied and adequate supply of food were essential elements that promoted the recovery of its patients. Good ventilation within the wards and wide avenues between the buildings made Chimborazo feel and smell much less like a hospital than would have been the case had it been housed in an old building in the heart of Richmond. Its location outside Richmond contributed to the peace and quiet needed for recuperation and allowed tighter enforcement of that quality when necessary.

Its proximity to Richmond also gave it many benefits. Chimborazo was close enough to allow McCaw to ride into town and receive an immediate answer from the surgeon general or medical director on a matter when needed. McCaw and his surgeons lived in Richmond and were placed on many medical boards. As part of the examining board for surgeons and assistant surgeons, McCaw was aware of the medical knowledge of the physicians who came before the board. His position and influence perhaps made it possible for him to request that certain talented medical officers be assigned to openings at Chimborazo, although no official documents show such requests. At the very least, he was able to choose some physicians among the many who sought positions at Chimborazo.

Another advantage of McCaw's hospital's size and location was its easy access to specialists who could deal with particularly difficult cases or provide special treatment. One day each week a dentist came to Chimborazo to perform any necessary dental work or operations. The dentist assigned to Chimborazo was Dr. W. Leigh Burton; he was given the rank of hospital steward.[4] In early 1865 Carrington directed McCaw to transfer cases of fracture of the superior or inferior maxillary bones to a special ward in the Receiving and Way Hospital for special treatment with a device known as Bean's Apparatus. "The apparatus . . . has been used with great success. It is constructed, adjusted and used by the Surgeon in attendance, aided by a Dentist, the inventor. [It] consists of any of the usual bandages for support of the lower jaw with strips of gutta precha between the teeth. These strips are moulded in impressions of the teeth and are vulcanized."[5] Also, as the war continued, groups of patients of "unsound mind" were transferred away from normal Confederate hospitals and placed in a separate facility.[6]

Although its physical characteristics and location provided many benefits to Chimborazo, perhaps its greatest advantage was its access to the most recent medical knowledge. The close connections that the hospital had with the Medical College of Virginia, the Association of Army and Navy Surgeons, and the *Confederate States Medical and Surgical Journal* all allowed Chimborazo's physicians to stay well informed about the latest medical ideas and treatments. An examination of the most common medical problems of the Civil War era and their corresponding treatments at Chimborazo and similar hospitals illustrates the level of medical knowledge at that time and the lively debate and exchange of information that surrounded medical treatment.

First of all, the hospital had a very close relationship with the Medical College of Virginia (MCV), at which McCaw held a faculty position. After March 1862 the MCV was the only medical school in the Confederacy to remain open. During the war the enrollment of the MCV increased to 228 students.[7] Chimborazo's connection to the medical school contributed to the hospital's status and placed it on the cutting edge of current medical treatments. McCaw encouraged the medical officers and stewards at Chimborazo to attend lectures there if they wished. This practice allowed medical officers to increase their knowledge on a variety of subjects and allowed stewards, many of whom were medical students, to continue their studies while receiving practical experience in a medical environment through their jobs at the hospital. Moore explained, "[A] certain number of young gentlemen were annually appointed hospital stewards, with the privilege of attending lectures at the Medical College of Virginia, and on graduation, letters of invitation were issued them for examination for appointment in the corps."[8] Evidently, Carrington also supported the connection. In one of his letters, he gave information about a series of lectures on military and operative surgery and explained that there would be no charge for medical officers or stewards to attend the lectures, except that the class would pay the costs to obtain the subjects of dissection and surgery. That particular class, taught by surgeon Charles Bell Gibson, met at one o'clock on Mondays, Wednesdays, and Fridays from April 1 to September 1, 1864.[9] Obviously, an emphasis on continued medical training remained a priority for the Confederate Medical Department and McCaw. The Medical Department had arranged for the lectures to be available, and McCaw was willing to let his medical staff go into town for quite a few hours every week.

The connection between Chimborazo and the MCV was not one-sided. Routinely, McCaw brought several medical students with him as he made rounds at his hospital. Also, some stewards who served at the hospital did so while they were students at the MCV. Records show that four of the six stewards serving at Chimborazo No. 4 in 1864 were attending lectures at the college. Several of these students worked at the hospital only when the MCV was in session.[10] Thus, Chimborazo became a teaching hospital for the most experienced surgeons and for the newest medical students. The variety of medical cases enhanced the students' medical education, and the presence of the students encouraged open-mindedness and thoughtfulness by Chimborazo's physicians. Even if absolutely no medical knowledge had been gained by the MCV students who made rounds with McCaw, their exposure to the hospital setting at Chimborazo and to McCaw's medical philosophy and management style doubtless affected their outlook and, through them, the subsequent development of hospitals in the American South.

Moore respected McCaw's clinical approach, which he illustrated by using Chimborazo as a source of information about medical drugs and treatments. On November 1, 1862, Moore sent McCaw a jug of medicine that John Asbell of Pulaski, Georgia, had sent to the Surgeon General's Office. Asbell started to use the medicine as a substitute for quinine, then discovered that it could cure "palpitation of the Heart." Asbell wanted to furnish the Confederate army with his medicine, but Moore first gave a sample of it to McCaw for "trial & report."[11] Although we do not know how Asbell's medicine did in its trial at Chimborazo, the surgeon general was evidently pleased with the quality of the study because several months later he asked for a similar trial to be run on the efficacy of "Worthington's Cholera Mixture."[12] The practice of using Chimborazo as a test facility became routine and continued throughout the war. Other examples of medicines tested were the Ointment of Podophyllin (a counter irritant recommended as a substitute for Croton Oil) and various expectorants, emetics, and demulcents (including Syrup Pruni Virginianae, Syrup Gillenia, Tinct. Sanguinana, Rad. Asclepius Tuberosa, Arium Tryphillum, and Vuls Gilenia). McCaw was to report not only on their general effectiveness but also "upon their uses,—specifically noting the forms of administration, and the combination and doses in which they prove most effectual."[13]

In 1864 Carrington wrote to McCaw with directions to set up a special study of "Camp Itch," a severe parasitic skin infection that Pember described as "that most hateful of all annoyances to the soldiers . . . that shirt of Nessus, which when once attached to the person clings there pertinaciously."[14] Carrington informed McCaw that all cases of skin diseases coming to Richmond that month would be sent to Chimborazo, mainly because of its "scientifically constructed baths." McCaw was ordered to set aside enough wards in his hospital to treat the skin diseases separately in order to determine "some general or specific methods of treatment that may be safe, speedy & not disagreeable." Carrington instructed McCaw to try "any plausible & well recommended mode of treatment." A report with Chimborazo's findings was to be sent to the medical director at the end of the month.[15]

Chimborazo's clinical emphasis and its reputation expanded even more at the end of the war through its connection with the *Confederate States Medical and Surgical Journal* (*CSMS Journal*), published from January 1864 to February 1865. The *CSMS Journal* served as one of the primary sources for information on medical topics in the South during the war. "Prior to the War, the South had no medical journal of more than local standing, and its physicians depended on Northern, British, and Continental journals," noted William D. Sharpe in his introduction to a reprinted compilation of issues of the journal.[16] In its first issue, the *CSMS Journal* stated its purpose:

> The Journal desires to be the representative of the profession, the exponent of its views, the record of its experience.
>
> Not only as the organ of the Southern medical profession, but as a means of imparting information to those who have, for three years, been debarred from any intercourse with the scientific world, will the publication of a medical periodical be found useful—indeed an absolute necessity. By taking advantage of the many opportunities to collect the recent literature of medicine . . . the editor hopes to render essential service to his readers, whilst with free access to the archives and reports of the Medical Department, and with the approval and under the supervision of the Surgeon-General, the vast statistics and tabulated records of the war can be carefully collated and made to subserve their legitimate uses. The task before us is arduous, the difficulties many, but if our brethren will give us an active and steady co-operation, success is not doubtful. We may have the proud satisfaction of believing that something has been done by us to advance and adorn the science to which our lives have been devoted, and with increased opportunities of knowledge we will be better able to do full justice to those whose lives are placed in our charge.[17]

The most obvious connection between Chimborazo Hospital and the *CSMS Journal* was through McCaw, who served as the major editor of the publication. McCaw's antebellum experience as an editor of several other medical journals no doubt prompted Moore to look to him when the idea of the journal began to be realized. Officially, Moore was given credit for the editorship, but quite a bit of evidence confirms McCaw as editor. For example, in November 1864 Carrington asked McCaw if he would be willing to publish "diagrams of Palmer's leg and arm, showing their internal construction, with descriptions of the same . . . and diagrams and descriptions of Bly's leg" in the journal.[18]

Not surprisingly, many of Chimborazo's medical officers stayed on top of new information and techniques through personal subscriptions to the journals.[19] However, a more important connection becomes obvious after a cursory glance at the contributors to the journal. Several of its medical officers—including all five of Chimborazo's surgeons-in-charge—wrote at least one article for the publication.

The *CSMS Journal* quickly gained the attention of the Confederacy's physicians. An editorial in the fifth publication stated that "Subscriptions have flowed in rapidly" and that the journal had "already attained a larger circulation than was ever reached before by any Southern medical periodical."[20] By the beginning of its second year, the editor reported, "The circulation of the Journal has surpassed any reasonable expectation, for such times as these surely do not favor the growth and cultivation of scientific studies."[21] Sadly, the journal suffered not from the lack of subscribers or the submission of items to print but instead from the shortage of paper and the difficulty that some mobile army physicians had in receiving the publication through the Confederate mail. The second problem decreased after an arrangement with the publishers allowed subscribers to prepay the postage of the journal through the Surgeon General's Office.

In his introduction to the reprinted *CSMS Journal*, Sharpe stated, "The level of the *Journal* is at least as high as that of its contemporaries, despite an extremely succinct style, although the quality of original material falls off in the last few issues. Original papers are for the most part case reports, statistical analyses and clinical lectures, some of which are models of their kind."[22] The journal received some attention outside the South, although most of the attention was centered around the journal's existence rather than on its scientific contributions. In 1864 the *Lancet*, published in London, reported that it had received several issues of the journal. The British journal praised the efforts of Southern physicians for their efforts to document and spread their knowledge and experience and specifically mentioned a couple of the articles printed in the journal.[23] Northern journals knew of the journal only through the *Lancet*, if at all. The *Cincinnati Lancet and Observer* mentioned the existence of the journal, as reported in the English journal, but an examination of thirteen other Northern medical journals yielded no mention or citation of the Confederate journal.[24]

Another feature of the *CSMS Journal* was its publication of the notes of the meetings of the Association of Army and Navy Surgeons of the Confederate States (AANS), which had been organized in August 1863. Invited by the faculty of the Medical College of Virginia and encouraged by the surgeon general, a large number of surgeons in Richmond and the surrounding area, including several at Chimborazo, met at the college to elect officers and begin the process of gathering and distributing information on many medical topics.[25] The group elected Moore as its president, McCaw as its vice president, and W. A. Davis, the surgeon-in-charge at Chimborazo No. 4, as its secretary.[26] The AANS's main goals, as stated in its constitution, were "the elucidation of practical and scientific points in the Military Surgery of this war, as illustrated by the individual experience of its members" and "to increase our information on subjects relating to Medical and Surgical Science by the accumulation of reliable data from the most authentic sources."[27] All Confederate surgeons and assistant surgeons could join the AANS by signing its constitution and paying annual dues of ten dollars.

The association held meetings every other week in Richmond on Saturday evenings, during which time its members read papers on medical topics, presented interesting cases they had encountered, and debated a variety of medical topics. As of January 1864 it was reported, "The debates of this Society have been attended with much interest, and have already eventuated in developing new channels of thought, and, in some respects, disclosed very unexpected and instructive results. . . . Reports of the conclusions arrived at . . . may reasonably be supposed to constitute hereafter no inconspicuous portion of the annals of this war."[28] Members not able to attend the meetings could contribute essays and papers to be read or pose questions for debate in their absence; if requested, replies to their questions would be returned via letter or telegraph to the corresponding members.[29] After January 1864 the *CSMS Journal* began publishing the minutes of the AANS meetings as a regular part of its contents.

Chimborazo's connections with the Medical College of Virginia, the *CSMS Journal*, and the AANS definitely contributed to the successful treatment of the hospital's patients. Through the records of the hospital and these other agencies, it is evident that medical treatment at Chimborazo both affected and was affected by the existing body of medical knowledge.

During its time of operation, Chimborazo Hospital admitted 77,889 patients. Patients were generally classified as sick, wounded, or convalescent. The registers show 50,350 admissions for specified sicknesses; 14,661 for wounds, accidents, or injuries; 771 as convalescents; and 50 as malingerers. The remaining 12,057 patients lacked a written diagnosis. Of the 23,849 cases with known results, 19,457 returned to duty, 677 were discharged, and 2,717 died. Thus, the mortality rate of Chimborazo hospital was 11.39 percent.[30]

One innovative feature of treatment at Chimborazo was its practice of distributing patients to different wards on the basis of their medical condition. In antebellum hospitals, the organization of patients in the wards rested on a first-come, first-serve basis. Hospitals typically only segregated men from women and whites from blacks. Administrators made few other distinctions, which led to higher death rates among patients. Separation by different types of illness was non-existent except for quarantining extremely contagious cases during an epidemic. Sometimes, patients with an unfamiliar collection of symptoms were admitted without a diagnosis. The lack of understanding about how disease spread compounded the problem, and many patients who entered a hospital for one malady soon had another to deal with as well.

Even at the beginning of the war, most hospitals tried to separate obviously contagious patients from the rest. This isolation was much more difficult in the smaller hospitals that had less room. Hospitals such as Chimborazo, with their separated wards placed in a pavilion design, were ideally suited for this problem. Ward A of each of Chimborazo's divisions was set aside to isolate contagious cases. Also, isolation tents were used for cases of erysipelas, pyaemia, and gangrene. Separate tents were pitched as needed to quarantine patients with smallpox, rubella, and other contagious illnesses; these tents held patients until they could be transferred to Howard's Grove Hospital. If a large number of patients contracted a contagious disease or infection within a short period, Ward A or a larger tent was used; smaller Sibley tents were used for isolating one or two patients. Using tents for contagious patients worked well, since they could easily be burned if required when they were no longer needed.

In addition to separating patients needing isolation, Chimborazo began the practice of separating patients on the basis of their medical diagnosis. This was relatively easily done, since most patients were transferred to the hospital in groups of either sick, wounded, or convalescent. Surgeon S. E. Habersham, in charge of Chimborazo No. 2, ordered sick and convalescent patients sent to Wards H, K, and L, designating his other twelve wards for wounded men.[31] Chimborazo's separation of patients by diagnosis categories made it easy for groups of patients to be transferred to hospitals in Lynchburg or other overflow areas to make room for wounded patients coming in from the battlefield. Chimborazo's early records indicate many instances in which an administrator from another hospital would inform McCaw that he had room for a certain number of patients at his facility. Once the divisions of the larger hospitals such as Chimborazo were designated to treat patients from particular states and most of the small hospitals had closed, the request for transfers based on state largely disappeared. However, for the first years of the war, separating patients by state and ailment when they arrived greatly facilitated finding groups of patients to transfer to other hospitals.

Convalescent patients were routinely kept apart from the sick and wounded. Most convalescents had chronic ailments and did not require constant attention. Instead, they mainly needed a nourishing diet and time to recuperate. Convalescent patients would neither be eligible for furlough nor be subject to transfer to other hospitals, but they could be detailed for light duty if their condition permitted. They could also be called by the military authorities to help defend the city if needed. In the summer of 1864, Carrington instructed McCaw that all of Chimborazo's convalescents should be immediately brought before an examining board and reevaluated to see if any could possibly return to duty. Since Chimborazo's physicians could not possibly examine all one thousand convalescent patients, General Robert E. Lee sent a board of medical officers for the task.

At times, when Chimborazo's regular wards became filled, the slightly wounded and sick could, as needed, be temporarily transferred to the convalescent tents to make room for the more critical patients. In mid-1864, in response to the high demand for room for new patients, administrators at Chimborazo requisitioned a hundred tents to form a convalescent division. Until the tents arrived, some convalescents had to bivouac around the hospital. In some of the secondary literature on Chimborazo, the hospital is reported to have had six divisions. The only explanation for the sixth would be a convalescent division, although primary sources do not record any reference to a formal sixth division.[32] Another practical reason for the separation of patients was convenience of treatment. Physicians treated patients' symptoms as they developed. If most of the patients in a ward were being treated for stomach or intestinal illnesses, then a supply of the medications that were routinely given could be kept conveniently on hand. A grouping of patients by ailment could also contribute to the knowledge and experience of the medical staff assigned to that ward; common symptoms and dangerous complications could be more easily recognized and effective treatments more easily determined.

Still another reason for the separation of patients was to study a particular group or a specific treatment given to a group. In March 1864 Surgeon-in-Charge W. A. Davis ordered, "[A]ll patients in this Division affected with disease of the skin will be transferred to Division No. 1."[33] Late in the war, Carrington directed McCaw to "have all men [patients and detailed men] disabled by ulcers of the lower extremities in each Division placed together in a ward and appropriately treated."[34] The patients were to be kept in bed and treated with Smith's anterior splints for a month, at the end of which a report to Carrington on the success or failure of the treatment was due. Smith's anterior splint was an easily made, simple, lightweight splint that used suspension from the ceiling. It worked well when properly used, but improper use could result in severe problems for the patient. This kind of study could determine the true value of the splint when properly used.[35]

Before the war hospitals rarely had enough patients with the same illness or set of symptoms to consider this option. As Bonnie Blustein noted, "Even where institutions had enough patients to make specialized wards feasible, 'specialism' was still suspect and attending physicians were under the watchful eyes of lay managers usually suspicious of research. The Civil War hospitals thus offered . . . an opportunity for clinical research almost unprecedented."[36]

Even though physicians liked the convenience of separation based on medical condition, in some ways separating patients who came from the same company could be difficult in terms of morale. In an unfamiliar hospital setting, men wanted to be close to their friends for companionship and protection. However, it also could hurt morale if, for example, one patient had a hearty appetite and was being served a full diet, while the patients around him were placed on restricted diets because of nausea or severe diarrhea.

As the war continued, the separation of patients using broad categories became more standard at Chimborazo and throughout the Confederacy. By mid-1863 the surgeon general required hospitals to establish a convalescent ward and a ward for contagious diseases.[37] Medical regulations for the following year extended that practice, directing that patients be "distributed according to the nature of their complaints."[38] Minimum compliance required the separation of convalescents, patients with diseases of the skin, eye, and ear, and the isolation of contagious cases.

One practical concern that hampered physicians' efforts to separate patients on the basis of ailment during the winter months was the lack of fuel and stoves. Patients had to be kept warm, and often that meant combining the different categories of patients into the same wards. The lack of fuel became a serious concern for Chimborazo during the winters of 1863 and 1864, even though there was money in its hospital fund to purchase fuel when it could be found. The fact that Chimborazo could still obtain some fuel prompted Medical Director Carrington to send all of the sick and wounded from Howard's Grove Hospital and from General Hospital No. 1 to Chimborazo in January 1864. These patients were to be kept in a separate division for several months—until the weather warmed sufficiently for them to return to the other facilities. Carrington informed McCaw that the beds in the division would not be needed for incoming transfers of other sick or wounded patients at least until April, when he estimated that the troops would begin their spring campaigns.[39] Although the intent to separate patients by illness seems common in the hospital correspondence, an examination of the hospital's patient registers shows a variety of patients admitted to some wards that were probably similar to today's medical-surgical wards. Evidently, many factors—including severity of illness, possibility of contagion, medical treatment, administrative processing, and available supplies—were considered by medical officers as they assigned patients to various wards.

The separation of patients by medical ailment was but the first step in treatment. Civil War physicians faced great challenges when dealing with their patients' medical problems. They saw and evaluated the medical conditions from a perspective distinctly different—and in many respects, backward—when compared to today's perspective. They practiced medicine reactively, based only on the symptoms that developed, instead of proactively, based on clinical findings.

In the search for understanding the causes of diseases, Civil War physicians remained baffled. There were no theories about bacteria or viruses. Some physicians and scientists had seen small objects under their microscopes, but they did not understand their differences or significance. The germ theory of disease was still far from the minds of physicians, much less ordinary Americans. The modern laboratory approach to medicine that identifies a specific microorganism as the specific cause for a specific disease was not only an unfamiliar process in the early to mid-nineteenth century but also an almost completely alien concept. Robert Koch's postulates, which explained the method for determining the specific microbial cause of a disease, was a revolutionary process even in 1884. Koch was a German scientist who, through carefully conducted studies of anthrax, formulated what are now known as "Koch's postulates," which prove that specific microorganisms cause specific diseases. Koch's postulates include the ideas that an organism must be present in animals suffering from the disease but must not be present in healthy animals and that it must be possible to induce the disease in a healthy animal using only the specific microorganism. Koch's work was instrumental in the development of microbiology and the development of medicine, because it stressed the importance of laboratory cultures.[40]

Antebellum physicians were not yet ready for Koch's ideas, but in the years before the war, an increased curiosity and open-mindedness about the mechanism of disease was evident. In the 1850s, as John Harley Warner has documented, quite a few American physicians had traveled to France to supplement their medical training, and while there they were influenced by the empiricism of French medicine, "exemplified by direct observation of symptoms in the living body and pathological lesions in the deceased."[41] Many of the Americans who returned from studying in France eventually became the elite in America's medical community and spread the approach of empiricism by contributing to medical journals and teaching in medical schools. According to Charles Rosenberg, "The Paris Clinical School—as it has come to be called by historians—crystallized a new way of looking at disease and of investigating it."[42] Instead of disease being seen as a general condition of the body, it was understood as a specific problem. The concept of specificity prompted physicians to investigate using an empirical approach to diagnose and classify different diseases. However, they worked using specificity of symptoms—not specificity of cause. "This way of working outwards *from* the cause *to* the symptoms and pathology (rather than in the other direction) has had significant effects on the classification of diseases—that is, on what conditions count as what disease."[43]

Instead of the modern practice of using symptoms to suggest tests that pinpoint the cause of the disease, Civil War physicians identified a disease by its symptoms and its course. American physicians and citizens thought a particular disease could result from a variety of causes. Those could be predisposing causes (the season or the constitution of the patient), external causes (the quality of the air around a patient or of his food), antecedent causes (some obstruction within the body), and immediate causes (a particular state of the blood).[44] All of the certainty that medical professionals now have, of at least knowing exactly what they are dealing with, was completely unfamiliar to the physician at Chimborazo. Physicians based their diagnosis of a patient on his symptoms, then based treatment on the attempt to halt the progression of the disease and comfort the patient by treating the symptoms. When a patient experienced several different medical problems, surgeons could become doubtful about which type of treatment would be most effective.

The development of secondary infections and the spread of infections to other parts of the body were very problematic to the physician trying to make sense of disease. "Not only did a pre-[laboratory] disease not have a specific causal agent, but it was possible to have 'mixed' diseases. It was also the case that diseases were considered capable of transforming into other diseases during their course."[45] If the familiar pattern of symptoms deviated from the norm, physicians could find themselves back at square one. Keeping good clinical records might help, but these could be incomplete because most physicians rarely noted the expected symptoms, especially those of diseases they dealt with every day, but instead documented the uncharacteristic symptoms. This practice could become confusing, given the large numbers of patients whom Confederate doctors treated and who had similar diseases; this was one reason why the Confederate Medical Department encouraged keeping records on all patients.[46]

Fortunately, the complex and unusual cases prompted physicians to keep an open mind when determining diagnosis and treatment. Physicians sought to understand the diseases, wounds, and infections that challenged them, but if a technique or medication worked, they used it—regardless of whether they understood how it worked. If the patient's health was strong enough, the common trial-and-error approach often hit on the right treatment eventually and helped the patient to recover. At times, even when Confederate physicians knew exactly which drug should be used, a shortage of that item might force another round of trial and error. Through practical experience and a growing understanding about disease, they often learned that their old methods did not work. This was explained in an article by Dr. John Hughes Bennet that McCaw published in the *CSMS Journal*. In "The Natural Progress of Disease," Bennet stated that the old practices of bloodletting, purging, antimony, and low diet to combat the spread of inflammation were known to be erroneous: "[T]he antiphlogistic treatment . . . not only fails to [cut short inflammations], but constitutes a most fatal practice."[47] Bennet blamed the error on "unacquaintance with the natural progress of disease," explaining, "Most diseases in vigorous constitutions . . . have a marked tendency to get well of themselves; whilst instead of loss of blood, weakness, and prostration being remedies, they are the sources of danger and the chief causes of the fatal result."[48] In the absence of a new pattern of treatment, physicians had learned to let the body heal itself and to intervene only when the benefits of treatment clearly outweighed the dangers.

Even though Civil War physicians were greatly hindered by their lack of understanding about how disease spread, their focus on empirical methods served them well. In contrast to the incompetence portrayed by many critics of Civil War medicine, the medical practices of the war as documented in Chimborazo's case record, the *CSMS Journal*, and in the *Medical and Surgical History of the Civil War* (the official multivolume account of medical practices during the war) were medically sound. The treatment of disease and infection changed during the war but did so on such a practical level that it did not seem obviously significant to medical historians. Through a trial-and-error technique practiced on hundreds and thousands of patients, physicians learned what medications and physical treatments worked best for a variety of medical problems.

The major medical problem of the Civil War—disease in its various forms—developed mainly from the living conditions of soldiers in the field. Personal and camp hygiene were greatly neglected, which compounded the large numbers of insects and vermin in the camps. Food that was insufficient in quantity and variety, as well as improperly cooked by soldiers, added to the problem. A lack of fresh water and properly placed and maintained latrines contributed as well. Soldiers suffered from exposure from living in tents and making long marches, especially during the latter years of the war when there was a lack of proper clothing, shoes, and blankets to protect them from the weather and the elements. All of these factors, combined with continued contact with large numbers of strangers from different regions, weakened the general health of the troops and almost assuredly resulted in sickness of some form or degree.[49]

When dealing with disease, an unglamorous but major part of Civil War medicine, physicians quickly learned the importance of hygiene. Far fewer cases of typhoid, diarrhea, and dysentery developed in camps led and populated by regular army, because those camps were typically cleaner. Epidemics ravaged camps with poor sanitation habits. Physicians in the North and the South quickly recognized this and tried to persuade medical officers that clean men, fresh water, properly cooked food, and the proper disposal of waste could make an enormous difference when calculating the number of men from their regiments who were healthy enough to fight. In the North the importance of this information and the incompetence in areas of the Union Medical Department prompted the formation of the United States Sanitary Commission and similar organizations. Over the course of the war, these groups greatly contributed to the effectiveness of the Union Medical Department and the general health of the Union troops. No such organizations were formed in the Confederacy, which lacked the networking, wealth, and civic spirit of the North. The effort in the South was spearheaded by the Confederacy's medical officers. Some regimental surgeons had difficulty convincing their troops and commanders of the importance of good sanitation and the value of enforcing measures to ensure clean camps. Confederate medical officers quickly determined that even if the soldiers' camps were unhealthy, the hospitals—obviously within their jurisdiction—would not be. At hospital posts such as Chimborazo, the commander ordered the camp's guard unit to enforce sanitation regulations.

Due to poor sanitation, poorly cooked food, and the open nature of camp life, illness among soldiers remained common throughout the war. When a soldier's sickness grew to an intolerable level, he reported for sick call for treatment by his regimental surgeon, who provided medications or admitted him to the regimental hospital. If the illness escalated, or if it continued long enough to require long-term treatment or recuperation, the surgeon ordered the patient transferred to a general hospital. Transfers of groups of patients from regimental to general hospitals commonly occurred when epidemics of various diseases went through a camp.

Most sick patients could be classified according to illnesses in one of five areas: gastrointestinal disorders, dietary deficiencies, fevers, pulmonary disorders, and skin irritations. Although these categories seem to include numerous illnesses, some of which will be mentioned separately, the classification of diseases during the nineteenth century before the isolation of the microorganisms that caused the specific ailments remained rather vague and often depended as much on the severity of the symptoms as on the specificity of the symptoms. When a patient had symptoms in several categories, the written diagnosis in the patient register normally reflected the condition that seemed most severe or life-threatening.

The most common category of sickness, not surprisingly, was gastrointestinal disorders—namely diarrhea and dysentery. The *Medical and Surgical History of the Civil War* introduced its lengthy report on these illness with the following statement:

> These disorders occurred with more frequency and produced more sickness and mortality than any other form of disease. They made their appearance at the very beginning of the war, . . . [and] were not long in acquiring a formidable character. Soon no army could move without leaving behind it a host of the victims. . . . In the general hospitals they were often more numerous than the sick from all other diseases, and rivalled the wounded in multitude.[50]

The remarks of a Confederate surgeon, Joseph Jones, supported that sentiment. "Chronic diarrhoea and dysentery were the most abundant and most difficult to cure amongst army diseases; and whilst the more fatal diseases, as typhoid fever, progressively diminished, chronic diarrhoea and dysentery progressively increased. . . . [M]ore soldiers were permanently disabled and lost to the service from these diseases than from the disability following the accidents of battle."[51]

Confederate statistics for 1861 and 1862 for troops located east of the Mississippi reported 226,828 cases of diarrhea or dysentery, making these maladies responsible for 26.7 percent of all reported cases of sickness. At Chimborazo alone, physicians diagnosed 10,503 patients with one of these maladies as their primary illness.[52] The statistics for the Union army's cases of diarrhea and dysentery numbered 1,739,135 cases with 44,558 deaths.[53] However, even as large as these numbers appear, they do not even approach the actual number of cases.[54] Another indicator of the importance of diarrhea and dysentery is obvious from a cursory glance at the contents of the *Medical and Surgical History of the Civil War*: two complete volumes, or 842 pages, are devoted to their recording and discussion.

The common symptom of both maladies was severe cramping and thin and frequent stools. From a clinical perspective, acute diarrhea was distinguished from acute dysentery by the absence of tenesmus (painful expulsive efforts) and fever, and from the greater occurrence of general nausea and vomiting.[55] The difference between chronic diarrhea and chronic dysentery was less obvious. Both illnesses progressed beyond the acute into a debilitating phase that might last for several months or longer. Many convalescent patients suffered from the "chronic" forms of the illnesses.

The causes of diarrhea and dysentery were myriad and mirrored the causes of illness in general that plagued the Union and Confederate armies. The treatments were even more varied, but some similarities did emerge. Most physicians began treatment by ordering rest and a bland diet that could be entirely digested in the stomach and upper intestines so as not to irritate the colon. Various medications were initiated to treat symptoms as they arose. "Hospital prescription books," Cunningham noted, "reveal that 'Blue Mass,' 'Astrgt Pills,' and 'Diarrhoea mixture' were some of the remedies most frequently prescribed."[56] Other treatments for the frequent bowel movements ranged from bromine to various popular indigenous astringents to nitrate of silver injections to the cauterization of the mucus membrane of the rectum. If one medication or treatment did not work, then physicians tried another and then another. Opiates were given for any severe pain experienced by patients.

One factor that made diarrhea so difficult to treat was its prevalence as a symptom of other maladies. Cunningham quoted one Confederate doctor as saying, "No matter what else a patient had . . . he had diarrhoea."[57] This quotation also reflects another problem with diarrhea. Because of the poor sanitary conditions in which soldiers lived, it remained so common that even when a patient recovered from the disorder, it might quickly return. Even in the hospitals, the lack of hand-washing could easily spread the condition.

The lack of a good diet among Confederate troops also contributed to the widespread occurrence of scurvy. Cunningham believed that incipient scurvy was misdiagnosed many times during the Civil War as diarrhea, dysentery, or debility—all very common diseases that resulted in numerous furloughs.[58] By 1863 scurvy became a big problem for the Army of Northern Virginia. In addition to affecting the general health of the troops, scurvy could also result in night blindness. "Lee's soldiers remembered seeing 'men led by the hand all night . . . go into battle with the command in the morning.'"[59] A proper diet restored sight and the patient's general health. Of the many thousands of patients admitted to Chimborazo, only 119 had diagnoses of scurvy.

The category of fevers was subdivided into continued fevers (such as typhoid), malarial fevers, and eruptive fevers. Eruptive fevers included smallpox, measles, erysipelas, and any other illness that combined a high fever with a skin rash. Many of these fevers subsided spontaneously after several weeks in healthy victims, but if they attacked a person with poor general health, or if a secondary infection or complication developed while the patient's health was compromised, they could become quite dangerous. Aware of that fact, physicians sought to keep the patient comfortable and to keep his general health as strong as possible while the primary illness ran its course. Common in the treatment of all fevers by Civil War physicians was the employment of cold sponges and other physical measures to bring the fever down, opiates given for restlessness, and a nourishing diet to help the patient retain his strength. Adequate fresh air and ventilation were also seen as critical features of treatment and containment, since physicians believed that the fevers spread through miasmas that came from current victims or unhealthy places. This miasmatic theory seemed to explain why cases of malaria (a parasitic infection now known to be spread by mosquitoes) and typhoid fever (a bacterial infection spread by contaminated water and flies) erupted in cycles and were more common in particular areas.

With regard to drug treatments, physicians, then as now, prescribed quinine to treat malaria. As the war continued and quinine became less available, physicians used turpentine—a popular substitute—or various native remedies, usually made from tree barks. The problem of obtaining quinine was heightened by the fact that malaria was normally treated in the camp and regimental hospitals, where shortages were the most severe because of the mobility of the facilities. Patients with malaria usually came only to general hospitals when complications or debility had severely compromised their health.[60] By the end of the war, quinine was being used not only as a treatment for malaria but also as a prophylactic in malaria-prone areas when it could be obtained by medical officers.[61]

One of the most severely feared fevers was smallpox, or variola. When a patient at Chimborazo developed smallpox, physicians immediately isolated him from the other patients until he could be transferred to the Howard's Grove Hospital, the Richmond hospital designated in 1863 to treat all military smallpox cases in the area. Howard's Grove was set up in the same way as any other pavilion hospital. Ward A was for the most contagious cases; Wards B and C were for lesser cases; Wards E and F were for patients recovering from smallpox but still having problems with other illnesses or wounds; and Ward D was set aside mainly for rubeola patients. Patient transfers from Howard's Grove usually occurred only out of Ward E. The three categories of variola listed in the patient registers were variola distinct, variola confluent, and variola malignant confluent. Among the patients treated at Howard's Grove were some officers and a few citizens. Not surprisingly, the death rate at Howard's Grove was quite high.[62]

After a smallpox patient left Chimborazo, the ward was thoroughly cleaned, disinfected, and aired, "and every precaution taken."[63] Any patients who had been recently exposed to smallpox, either in the field or the hospital, were not granted leaves of absence, furloughs, or transfers to hospitals other than those set aside for smallpox cases.[64] Even with the strict policies, however, some physicians at other hospitals evidently did not understand how easily smallpox spread.

Surgeon W. A. Davis reported the arrival of Private M. G. Fitz, a patient who had been transferred from Howard's Grove back to Chimborazo: "His personal clothing (woolen) was brought with him: he states that it was taken directly from his bed in the Smallpox Hosp & forwarded without any purification. I have caused this man to be isolated, & have directed that all his clothing should be thoroughly cleansed. He is very feeble, & still bears upon his person the marks of recent variola."[65]

To prevent the spread of smallpox, the Medical Department attempted to vaccinate all soldiers who came through its hospitals. Throughout the war, the Medical Department routinely circulated orders, reminding medical officers of their duty to comply fully with vaccination policy. An 1863 circular from the Surgeon General's Office provided medical officers with specific instructions on vaccinating with the scab and with the lymph to ensure that vaccinations were being done properly. The circular instructed, "The best instrument for [vaccinating with the scab] is an old lancet, with the point broken off. . . . [T]he lancet cannot then (as it ought never to) be used for any other purpose."[66] Before any soldiers could be returned to duty, the medical officer of their ward had to provide the hospital's clerk with a list of those who had been vaccinated.[67] A personalized ticket was given to each soldier who left the hospital with information about when he had been vaccinated or revaccinated, the type of vaccination used, and the hospital from which he had come. When he returned to his company, the surgeon-in-charge there took his ticket before allowing him to rejoin his unit. To further ensure compliance of the practice, field surgeons were required to report the names of hospitals that were disobeying regulations by not providing the necessary tickets.[68]

One problem with vaccinations was that much of the vaccine was inert. Even if the physician performed the procedure correctly, the vaccine had to be strong enough to inoculate the patient; otherwise, it might as well have never been done. H. H. Cunningham noted, "A record of 307 vaccinations in one of the divisions of Chimborazo Hospital during the months of June and July, 1864, . . . showed the number 'taken' to have been 134 and the number 'not taken' to have been 173."[69] An article in the *CSMS Journal* explained that the presence of a scab validated the effectiveness of the vaccination. If the virus used to vaccinate was inert or defective in some way, either no scab or an "imperfect one" would result.[70]

Surgeon General Moore used the lack of potent vaccine to justify the practice of immunizing Southern children.[71] In February 1864 the Surgeon General's Office instructed the medical directors of hospitals "to promptly assign one Assist Surg in each of the larger cities of the Confederacy to the temporary & special duty of vaccinating gratis, in such cities & precincts, all healthy children, white & black, who have not been previously vaccinated."[72] Vaccine made from human scabs, especially those from children, was believed to be the most effective. Thus, if a large number of Confederate children had been immunized successfully, it would not only have benefited the health of the general public but would also have provided a large pop-ulation from which to obtain scabs to make vaccine for the troops. The order reveals that the Surgeon General's Office had, at least on a limited scale, begun concerning itself with the health of the general public as well as that of the army, even if it had an ulterior motive. This extension of military medicine into the civilian sector was extremely uncommon in the nineteenth century, when the federal government nor-mally did very little in any area of private life, including public health.

Because of the fear surrounding smallpox and its easy spread, early and accu-rate diagnosis was critical. An unexpected diagnosis technique was reported in an article by surgeon J. C. M. Merillat in the May 1864 issue of the *CSMS Journal*. Merillat, who was stationed at the General Hospital at Staunton, Virginia, con-ducted a daily urine analysis using a test tube and nitric acid and reported on his observations and techniques concerning how to distinguish smallpox from rube-ola. He concluded, "[T]he chlorides are never present in the urine during the two first stages of smallpox. . . . [T]he quantity of the chlorides in the urine of patients laboring under rubeola is normal during the whole progress of that disease."[73] The most significant feature of Merillat's contribution does not concern the diagnosis of the two diseases but the fact that he was using a chemical analysis of urine as his method, which strongly indicates the attempt, at least, of a laboratory ap-proach to diagnosis. Merillat was by no means the first to do a chemical analysis of urine—it was a common practice in parts of Europe. However, it is surprising that this analysis would be done at a Confederate army hospital in western Virginia. Thus, the process was apparently becoming widespread. Also significant is the fact that Merillat conducted the analysis of these patients' urine on a daily basis. At the end of his article, he pointed out his inability to obtain a microscope with high magnifying powers but added, "I have found one magnifying 100 lin-ear diameters sufficient for [the purpose of making observations on the urine in different diseases]."[74]

Among the pulmonary and respiratory diseases commonly treated during the Civil War were pneumonia, pulmonary tuberculosis, pleurisy, catarrh, and bron-chitis. The unavoidable conditions of exposure that military troops faced explain the large numbers of soldiers who suffered from these conditions.[75] Unfortunately, Confederate soldiers seemed to have had more trouble with respiratory ailments than their Northern counterparts. One explanation for this was the lack of ade-quate clothing, blankets, and supplies that challenged the Confederacy's troops. Another possible reason relates to the shortage of manpower in the South, which resulted in fewer discharges of patients with persistent respiratory problems. Instead of granting discharges, according to the *Medical and Surgical History*, "the policy of [the Confederate] government was to hold every man for such duty as he could perform."[76]

As the *Medical and Surgical History* also related, the most serious of these ill-nesses was pneumonia:

> Many diseases were of more frequent occurrence than pneumonia,
> but only diarrhoea and dysentery and the continued fevers furnished
> a larger death-list. It has been shown, however, . . . that pneumonia
> was present and caused or hastened the fatal issue in 21.6 per cent of
> the deaths from diarrhoea and dysentery and in 68.3 per cent of those
> contributed to the continued fevers; the mortality from measles also
> resulted largely from inflammatory processes in the lungs. In fact, the
> importance of pneumonia as a destroyer of life in our camps and
> hospitals can hardly be overestimated.[77]

Physicians had long believed pneumonia to be an inflammation of the lungs and therefore treated their antebellum pneumonia patients with heroic depleting mea-sures, such as the use of antimony and bleeding, to decrease the amount of inflam-mation. This treatment, however, did not work with the already weakened soldiers with whom Civil War doctors dealt.

Recognizing their failed methods, many physicians adjusted their approach and ordered treatment that might help alleviate the pneumonia patient's fever without diminishing his general strength. "[G]eneral depletion was rarely em-ployed as an antagonist to the febrile state," according to the *Medical and Surgical History.* "Medical officers recognized the adynamic influences that affected the troops and declined, in a disease which was so frequently fatal by asthenia, to pur-chase temporary relief at the expense of an impoverishment of an already deteri-orated blood."[78] Instead, physicians focused on supportive measures that would inhibit the extension of the inflammation, decrease the patient's suffering, and strengthen the general constitution. Usually, they prescribed small doses of tartar emetic, a mercurial drug, to allay fever and depress the inflammation; opiates, such as Dover's powder, to calm the patient and relieve pain; and syrups of vari-ous types to help relieve coughing.[79]

Modern physicians use antibiotics to treat the major cause of pneumonia, which is a bacterial infection. A patient's prognosis depends on his general health and the type of bacteria causing the infection. Although Civil War physicians obviously did not have access to antibiotics, their use of mercurial drugs, which are classified as anti-infectives, was on the right track. Antibiotics work by killing enough of the bacteria so that the body's natural defenses can gain the upper hand and take care of the rest. Anti-infectives work by making the body's environment less favorable for the microorganisms to reproduce, thus halting the increased numbers and at least giving the body's defenses a better chance to work. Although modern physicians have a wider variety of drugs at their disposal to treat the symptoms of pneumonia, the focus, then as now, was on treating the cause first and the symptoms and general condition of the patient second. The shift from the depleting treatments to the supportive ones—a very practical move prompted by careful observation and common sense—was instrumental in the effective treatment of the respiratory diseases.

Tuberculosis, then referred to as consumption, was another major respiratory disease. Although some consumptives seemed strengthened by the fresh air and rigors of field service, the lack of an adequate diet and the daily challenges to the immune system that all Civil War soldiers faced could easily result in the flare-up of the disease. A severe cough, producing large amounts of yellow or blood-streaked matter, pain in the upper part of the chest, and a frequent and feeble pulse marked the most common symptoms of tuberculosis. Lacking the specific drug treatments that modern physicians use, Civil War surgeons mainly treated the chronic illness with alcoholic stimulants, various tonics, and a nourishing diet to improve the patient's general strength. At night they used opiates to relieve restlessness and coughing.[80]

One interesting feature of medical practice also reveals itself when the trained medical professional examines the medical reports and cases of respiratory illness that were recorded by Civil War surgeons. Most historians have rejected the idea that Civil War surgeons routinely used stethoscopes, basing this assumption on the fact that very few medical schools utilized the instrument. However, Dr. George Banken, a physician who spoke in 1994 at the National Museum of Civil War Medicine, has discounted the theory. After a thorough examination of the *Medical and Surgical History,* he strongly believes that stethoscopes were widely used during the war. In numerous cases the physicians recorded hearing rales and distinguished which lobe of the lung the sounds were heard. Dr. Banken asserted that observations that specific could not be determined without the use of a stethoscope.[81]

The last major disease classification was that of skin disorders, of which "Camp Itch" was the most common. Although not life-threatening, itch seemed contagious, sometimes spreading through camps in epidemic-like fashion, affecting large numbers of soldiers. Most physicians from the North and South had never treated this condition before, although some western doctors recognized it, referring to it as prairie dog itch, western itch, Illinois Itch, or Missouri Mange. The skin inflammation differed from scabies, with which most physicians were familiar, because of its lack of a parasite. Itch generally attacked the arms, chest, abdomen, and lower extremities and began with the development of small, solid, elevated lesions that itched intolerably. Scratching and other irritation to the affected area caused the lesions to join together, grow crusty, and become filled with a thin, yellowish, acrid fluid. By this point, the inflammation was not only irritating but painful as well.

Doctors believed itch to originate from a combination of an unknown local irritant and an unhealthy environment. The routine treatment in the South was a sulfur, arsenic, or alkaline bath, but the difficulty of procuring the ingredients for such baths prompted physicians to turn to various other treatments for relief. The *CSMS Journal* included two such treatments in its issues. In the first, patients in the initial stages of the irritation were given a strong concoction of poke root (*Phytolacca decandra*) to bathe with twice a day, which they then washed off with soap and water. If the skin had already become inflamed, the poke root treatment caused too much pain, so physicians ordered a dedoction (extraction by boiling in water) of broom straw root or of slippery elm, given three or four times per day, until the inflammation subsided enough for the poke root to be used. The poke root treatment could also be administered as an ointment or dedoction. This botanical treatment was quite practical, because both poke and broom straw were very common field plants in Virginia.[82] Another reputable treatment was an ointment made of elder bark and sweet gum, which was applied to the affected area twice a day.[83]

Some cases of itch did develop to the point where the patients were admitted to a hospital. Several patients came to Chimborazo with the admitting diagnosis recorded as Camp Itch. Chimborazo's baths, located on the downslope of its plateau, made it a logical place for itch patients to be assigned.[84] Throughout the war, several studies were done at Chimborazo to determine the most effective remedies and treatments for the common skin irritation. Physicians at Chimborazo also reported on the effectiveness of the leaves and juice of the elder as a treatment for pediculi, lice, and chinchee.[85]

Although disease in its various forms affected the majority of patients admitted to Chimborazo and other Confederate hospitals, the treatment of wounds received an enormous amount of attention as well. At Chimborazo, wounded patients made up 14 percent of admissions up until late 1863, then almost 20 percent in the last two years of the war.[86] Most of these patients had been previously treated by army physicians in field hospitals before being transferred to Chimborazo by way of the Receiving and Way Hospital in Richmond. Therefore, they often arrived at Chimborazo several days after being wounded—sometimes in good condition, sometimes not. Phoebe Pember recorded an example of a soldier who arrived in horrible condition, which she described as the "most sickening" wounded case she encountered at Chimborazo. This soldier was part of a group of wounded who had not received medical treatment for three days because the railroad tracks to Richmond had been cut by Union soldiers. Pember continued:

He was taken into a ward, seated on a bed, while I stood on a bench to be able to unwind rag after rag from around his head. . . .

Two balls had passed through his cheek and jaw within half an inch of each other, knocking out the teeth on both sides and cutting the tongue in half. . . . There was nothing fatal to be apprehended, but fatal wounds are not always the most trying.

. . . The swollen lips turned out, and the mouth filled with blood, matter, fragments of teeth from amidst all of which the maggots in countless numbers swarmed and writhed, while the smell generated by this putridity was unbearable. Castile soap and soft sponges soon cleansed the offensive cavity, and he was able in an hour to swallow some nourishment he drew through a quill.[87]

When battles occurred near Richmond, some patients came to the hospital on the hill directly from the battlefield. When this was likely, Chimborazo's surgeons were put on alert. This is evident in an order issued by Dr. Habersham, surgeon-in-charge of Chimborazo No. 2:

The Medical Officers of this Division will hereafter remain in the Hospital until further orders from 9 AM to 1½ and from 4 to 7 PM. Strict obedience to this order is incumbent because of the large number of Wounded which will be daily sent to this Division. The Ward Surgeons will order their Ward Masters to report to them immediately the wounded received so that they may be seen and attended to immediately by the Ward Surgeons.[88]

As an interesting side note, Phoebe Pember wrote the following after a battle in the area: "There were not as many desperate wounds among the soldiers brought in that night as usual. Strange to say, the ghastliness of wounds varied much in the different battles, perhaps from the nearness or distance of contending parties."[89]

Injuries of the extremities made up the majority of wounds treated at Chimborazo. This was typical of wounded patients in any Confederate hospital. Dr. Julian J. Chisolm estimated in his authoritative *Manual of Military Surgery*, commissioned by Surgeon General Moore and published in 1863, that 65 percent of Confederate wounds were in the extremities.[90] Extremity wounds could take several months to heal. Generally, the farther the wound site was from the trunk, the better the chance of survival for the patient.

Wounds in other areas of the body were less frequent and more dangerous. Chisolm reported that 19 percent of wounds were chest wounds, 12 percent were in the head or neck, and less than 5 percent were in the abdomen.[91] Abdomen and chest wounds were frequently fatal since vital organs were commonly damaged. For this reason, soldiers wounded in those areas rarely made it out of the field hospitals. Field surgeons treated the wounded who had a better chance of surviving before they tackled the more severe cases that offered little hope.

Chimborazo received few patients with severe wounds, although records do reveal some exceptions. For example, the *CSMS Journal* reported a study of eleven cases of compound fracture of the cranium by gunshot wounds that were treated at Chimborazo.[92] While at the hospital, physicians kept detailed records of these cases. Interestingly, in the case of one of the patients, Private H. Dixon of North Carolina, the journal reported, "This case is one which would seem to have demanded the use of the trephine, but, guided by the experience of Stromeyer, McLeod, and other military surgeons of high reputation, it was decided not to operate. The entire recovery of this soldier justified the omission of the operation and the course of treatment that was pursued." Amazingly, only two of the eleven died; the rest recovered and were either returned to duty or were furloughed home.[93]

Surgeon P. F. Browne reported another example of an extremely serious wound treated at Chimborazo. Private J. W. Branson of Virginia received a gunshot wound to the chest that affected one of his lungs. When he arrived at Chimborazo less than twenty-four hours after the injury, surgeons there decided not to operate but instead created a hermetic or airtight seal around the wound. After several weeks, the patient recovered and was furloughed home to recuperate fully.[94] This case is noteworthy because it provides a specific example of Chimborazo as an excellent hospital, staffed with surgeons performing new treatments effectively. The new medical procedure, called "hermetically sealing," was first proposed by B. Howard, a U.S. assistant surgeon, in the *New York Medical Times* and reported in the fourth issue of the *CSMS Journal*. It encouraged physicians, when dealing with penetrating gunshot wounds of the chest or abdomen, to create an airtight seal over the entrance and exit wounds of the bullet. The full description of hermetically sealing included removing all accessible foreign bodies, converting the circumference of the wound into an elliptical form, trimming away all injured parts, suturing the wound, drying the surface, and securely cementing the wound with collodion (a solution of pryoxylin in ether or alcohol). This treatment, which allowed no air into the wound, controlled hemorrhage, relieved dyspnea, and prevented suppuration. The well-known Confederate surgeon J. J. Chisolm extended this idea to all gunshot wounds in the ninth issue of the *CSMS Journal*—an idea that was applauded by the journal's editor in the same issue.[95] The fact that the surgeons at Chimborazo tried this treatment and did so effectively reveals their efforts to think about their options of medical treatment instead of simply doing what had always been done. Surgeon Browne's published report of the treatment reveals his interest, as well as that of McCaw, in providing the Confederate medical community with documented evidence of the effectiveness of the new treatment.

Ninety-four percent of the wounds received in Civil War battles were inflicted by bullets—the most common of which was the minié ball. The minié ball was a conoidal-shaped, hollow-nosed, soft lead .58-caliber bullet that tended to flatten on impact.[96] Its low velocity frequently caused it to remain in soft tissue or to leave a large, bursting exit wound. "By making a large wound and carrying with it bits of skin and clothing, the bullet almost ensured infection. Its impact often shattered a section of any bone it encountered, leading to a high percentage of amputations."[97] A Confederate surgeon, Simon Baruch, noted, "The shattering, splintering, and splitting of a long bone by the impact of a minie . . . ball [was] in many instances, both remarkable and frightening."[98]

Some soldiers received several shot wounds in the same battle. Many of these unfortunate men died on the battlefield or soon after, but some did survive. Hospital reports recorded the injuries that seemed most severe. Multiple wounds, especially when more than one was severe, greatly decreased the chance of a full recovery. Union records revealed one soldier from Massachusetts, Private Franz Metzel, who "accidentally got between or in the range of cross-firing" and received twenty-six separate gunshot wounds at the Battle of Spottsylvania. He died twenty-eight days later at Armory Square Hospital in Washington.[99]

After receiving a gunshot wound, a soldier often experienced shock, pain, and a loss of blood. More severe wounds prompted more immediate and crippling symptoms. According to the *Medical and Surgical History*, "It is probable that a large percentage of the 'killed in battle' were cases where primary haemorrhage [*sic*] followed the division of important vessels, death ensuing instantly or before help could be procured."[100] Those who did not die quickly were treated by assistant surgeons in the primary stations near the battlefield or helped back to field hospitals for treatment. There, physicians conducted a full examination of the wound, using their fingers. The *Medical and Surgical History* reported, "This examination was generally conducted under the influence of anaesthetics for the purpose of accurate diagnosis; in its course, balls and foreign bodies were extracted, bleeding vessels secured, and splinters of bone removed; upon its conclusion such operations were performed as in the judgment of the surgeon were necessary."[101]

For severe wounds in the extremities, the decision about whether to amputate remained controversial. Early in the war, amputations were performed routinely by the young surgeons who had little surgical skill and a desire to gain experience. As the level of surgical knowledge and experience increased, a debate developed concerning amputation versus more conservative surgeries. The more conservative surgeons preferred resection (the cutting off of the head of a bone when shattered) and excision (removing part of the shaft of the bone) when at all possible, although the limb that remained was usually only partially useful, if at all. In the general consensus that developed, amputation was recommended when the limb's muscles were badly lacerated, when a fracture involved a joint, or when the bone was splintered. In such cases amputation was seen as not only justified but necessary to save the person's life. To investigate the matter, Moore requested information from the surgeons-in-charge of every hospital in Richmond, asking them to report "the number of cases of compound fracture of the thigh, [caused by gunshot] treated without amputation, and the result of said treatment in each case."[102] Statistics from Richmond hospitals strongly supported the use of conservative surgery instead of amputation: of 388 cases of gunshot wounds to the thigh, the recovery rate for patients treated with conservative surgery was almost 40 percent, while that of patients receiving amputations was less than 15 percent.[103] Overall, although excision probably worked well when performed by experienced surgeons in a stable environment, amputation worked best in the field hospitals when the large numbers of wounded required surgeons to perform operations on several hundred soldiers per day. Professor Skey, a surgeon at St. Bartholomew's Hospital, wrote the following about the debate in an article reprinted by the *CSMS Journal*: "[I]n all doubtful cases, I would give the benefit of the doubt to the patient, and endeavor to restore the limb."[104]

At Chimborazo, the decision about amputation also depended on the general condition of the patient. Sergeant B. B. Duke came to Chimborazo with a gunshot wound to his elbow joint that he had received at the Second Battle of Fredericksburg. Until he reached Chimborazo he had not received any medical or surgical attention. If a field surgeon had treated him, amputation would have resulted since the wound was so extensive. However, by the time he got to Chimborazo, he was so anemic and weak that the surgeons decided he probably would not survive the operation. When inflammation developed at the wound site, sedative lotions were applied, and anodynes and narcotics given to treat the pain. Several small incisions were made in the vicinity of the joint to evacuate the pus. The raised entrance and exit wounds were cautiously and carefully treated with silver nitrate.[105] This case provides one example of the conservative approach used by Chimborazo's surgeons, and it contrasts sharply with the popular image of Civil War surgeons' propensity to amputate.

To control bleeding, surgeons used ligatures, which soon replaced the tourniquets and cauterizing used early in the war. "The use of ligature and skill in applying them was one of the major advances in surgical technique," according to F. William Blaisdell.[106] When ligatures were used, hemorrhage—a major complication early in the war—rarely occurred except in cases of severely infected wounds. Commonly, ligatures were made of silk, although boiled horse hair and other materials were used in the Confederacy late in the war as shortages of supplies increased. Interestingly, these substitute ligatures often worked as well or better than the silk; the process of boiling the material before use to make it pliable actually sterilized it, prohibiting infection.

After the wound was treated, it was dressed simply with lint or linen and a rolled bandage and kept moist with cold water.[107] Patients with severe wounds were then transferred to a general hospital for further treatment and recuperation. In the hospitals the major treatment generally consisted of cleaning and dressing the wound once or twice a day and keeping the dressings cold. Cold-water dressings were seen as "invaluable in the treatment of gunshot wounds," according to Surgeon J. B. Read, who explained that the cold applications helped heal the wound by modifying and restraining inflammation. The cold water, Read wrote, could be applied "by direct application, dripping, and by applications covered [often with greased or oiled pieces of material] so as to prevent evaporation and exclude air."[108] The cold-water dressings perhaps also helped the swelling and fever that accompany a wounded site that is fighting off infection. White blood cells converge on the area to surround and consume the foreign organism. Swelling occurs as the number of white blood cells increases as needed. Fever generally occurs to increase the body's metabolism so that more white blood cells can be produced. If the body is not strong enough to fight off the microorganism, swelling and fever continue to escalate, and other symptoms develop as the microorganism multiplies and emits its toxins.[109]

The wounded area was then immobilized as much as possible to promote healing. Chimborazo's physicians commonly used Smith's anterior splint to immobilize leg wounds and prevent shortening of the limb. The lightweight wire splint, obtained through the medical purveyor, could be a blessing or a curse to patients, depending on how skilled their physician was in its use. Improper use could cause pain, abrasion, ulceration, and abscess. Because of this, and in response to the popular request for more information on the proper use of the apparatus, the *CSMS Journal* printed instructions in its May 1864 edition.[110]

Other than direct treatment of the wound, physicians focused on supportive measures to improve the general condition of the patient. For pain relief they ordered opium, morphine, and Dover's powder. To help fight infection, they ordered stimulants such as whiskey, brandy, and muriated tincture of iron. A nourishing diet of soups, chicken, eggs, bread and butter, milk, coffee, and eggnog, along with orders for rest and fresh air, rounded out the treatment.

The medical record of Sam Williams, a patient with a gunshot wound just below his knee, provides an example of common treatment in 1864. Williams was given tincture of iron three times a day and placed on a full diet with whiskey. His wound was treated with chlorine tincture and kept wet with water. Five days later, he began receiving quinine as well as iron, and turpentine was applied to the wound when dressed. Over the next several days, an elm poultice was also applied to the wound. Starting on July 11, the wound was completely irrigated during the day and a poultice placed on it during the night. However, the suppuration worsened and gangrene developed. Disinfectants were then ordered. Williams received opium for pain. During the last week of his treatment, his diet changed to "milk & rice," "spoon diet," and "beef tea diet," which reflected his general weakness. After a thirty-two-day stay at the hospital, he died on July 24. At that time his diagnosis read, "V.S. [Vulnus Sclopeticum, or gunshot wound] of knee with extensive suppurative and necrosis of head of tibia. Discharge very offensive, sore mouth & throat."[111] Williams's treatment seems to be typical. Wounds were treated with simple drip irrigation until symptoms of serious infection began to appear, at which time the doctors would order disinfectants.

The only surviving mortality numbers for Chimborazo Hospital's wounded patients were published in the *Confederate States Medical and Surgical Journal*. According to this source, from November 1, 1861, to November 1, 1863, the hospital had treated 6,740 cases of Vulnus Sclopeticum with 377 deaths—a 5.74 mortality rate.[112] If accurate, these numbers are amazingly low.

The most serious threat to a wounded patient was—and still is—infection. Common indications of an infection include inflammation at the infected site and general symptoms such as fever, chills, and malaise. If not treated quickly, the infection may break down the body's local defense barriers, allowing the infection to spread to other parts of the body via the bloodstream. During the Civil War, infection was almost certain to follow the infliction of a wound. Probing by dirty fingers and instruments and washing with common cloths and sponges with water from common pails were common practices. According to medical historians Julian E. Kuz and Bradley P. Bengtson, "Nearly all wounds became infected, and white, creamy 'laudable' pus was felt to be a good prognostic sign and part of the normal healing process. Wounds that healed without suppuration were essentially considered abnormal and were reported as curiosities."[113] One logical reason why laudable pus was viewed as good was that, in cases of gangrene or erysipelas, only minimal amounts of pus drained from the wound. Thomas Watson explained the common beliefs about inflammation and suppuration in his 1858 medical text: "It is through inflammation that parts adhere together . . . and that foreign or hurtful matters are conveyed safely out of the body."[114] When inflammation became aggravated and swollen and began to discharge pus, Watson wrote, "there generally ensues a considerable and speedy abatement of all the local symptoms of inflammation—the pain, the heat, the redness, the [swelling]."[115]

Added to the difficulty of fighting infection was the general condition of many soldiers when they were wounded. Men weakened by disease, malnutrition, and exhaustion had little hope against infection of any kind. A Union surgeon, J. S. Billings, wrote, "Operating, as I did, upon men whose vital force had been diminished by scorbutus and malaria, and exhausted by transfer from a distance, I had little hope of successful results."[116] When reviewing medical records from the Civil War, it is surprising that wounded patients fared as well as they did.

The first step modern physicians take to treat an infection is to isolate the specific microorganism that is causing the problem. Then, once they know their enemy and its specific characteristics, they are able to prescribe the appropriate medication and take any appropriate isolation measures to protect the medical staff, visitors, and other patients from infection. Without an understanding of how infection was caused, Civil War physicians waited until the symptoms of the infection began to worsen before they began to diagnose and treat it, which severely handicapped their efforts. As the *Merck Manual* points out, "Manifestations of infectious diseases are protean because infectious agents differ widely and may involve any organ system of the body. Furthermore, many manifestations result from nonspecific host responses rather than from direct actions of infecting organisms."[117]

Several distinct kinds of life-threatening infection therefore threatened the wounded soldier. Physicians, nurses, and patients quickly learned to fear the early characteristics of the four most feared infections: gangrene, erysipelas, pyemia, and tetanus. These infections killed many more men than was actually reported during the war, due to the nature of the hospitals' records. Accurate numbers are impossible to obtain since records provide only a patient's admitting diagnosis, such as "V.S. knee," and frequently do not record any further developments in its main registers. Thus, many patients who seemingly died from gunshot wounds may have actually died from the infections that developed in those wounds.

One of the greatest threats to a wounded patient was gangrene. Most gangrene cases—89.6 percent of the Union's recorded cases—developed in wounds in the extremities.[118] In many cases surgery (either an amputation or an excision) was performed because of the severity of the wound. Poor operating conditions in the makeshift field hospitals greatly contributed to the incidence of many types of infections—gangrene was only one very visible example. However, without basic aseptic techniques being observed, even operations performed in the established general hospitals such as Chimborazo could easily threaten a patient's life.

The distinctive offensive odor and horrifying appearance of a gangrenous wound caused fear even among those who were unfamiliar with the dangers of the infection. Civil War surgeons reported various types of gangrene in their reports of cases during the war. They tried to categorize the different types of the infection in an effort to better understand the differences in its progression. *The Medical and Surgical History of the Civil War* grouped these cases together, explaining, "According to the conception or predilection of the surgeon, these terms, in many instances, seem to have been used indiscriminately, and it has been found utterly impossible to determine with accuracy the cases of traumatic gangrene, hospital gangrene, dry gangrene, etc."[119]

"Hospital gangrene" was particularly feared because of its extremely fast progression. "This complication, in retrospect," noted William Blaisdell, "appeared to be a synergistic infection that was a combination of aerobes and anaerobes, such as *Streptococcus* combined with anaerobic gram-negative bacteria."[120] One surgeon wrote, "'Hospital gangrene, the typhus of wounds,' is, in its most marked form, a fearful and unwelcome guest in any hospital. . . . It claims many victims in its fierce attacks, and often puts to naught all the resources of the most skillful surgeon."[121] Kate Cumming, a Confederate matron who served in hospitals of the Army of Tennessee, wrote of an outbreak of hospital gangrene: "Our wounded are doing badly; gangrene in its worst form has broken out among them. Those whom we thought were almost well are now suffering severely. A wound which a few days ago was not the size of a silver dime is now eight or ten inches in diameter."[122] The quick spread of this infection seemed particularly insidious when the patients were kept in crowded, badly ventilated, or unclean areas. "It was also noticed that the incidence of hospital gangrene seemed 'to increase in proportion to the distance which the wounded were transported from the battlefield,'" H. H. Cunningham wrote.[123]

Fatigue, exposure, bad food, and other factors that decreased the general health of the troops also contributed to the development of gangrene and other infections in wounded patients, because the patients' bodies were less able to fight off the microorganisms. Because of this connection, some physicians, a minority, went so far as to argue that gangrene might be a constitutional instead of a local disease. In response to this debate, one Union surgeon noted that constitutional symptoms were not always present, and when they were, they usually remained slight, unlike the grave condition of the affected wound. He also wrote, "No one as yet has ever seen the disease *originate* constitutionally, but *always* locally. Wounds may become gangrenous; but hospital gangrene never gives rise to ulcers."[124] Logically, then, remedying the unclean conditions was essential to cure the patients affected with gangrene and to keep the problem from spreading to others.

Today's physicians know that gangrene (progressive myonecrosis) is a potentially lethal wound infection caused by clostridia, an anaerobic, spore-forming, gram-positive bacteria. According to the *Merck Manual,* "Infection develops hours or days after injury occurs, usually in an extremity after severe crushing or penetrating trauma that results in much devitalized tissue."[125] Modern treatment includes intravenously administered antibiotics, thorough wound debridement, and, if necessary, amputation of the affected extremity at least several inches above the inflamed area.

Civil War surgeons began to treat gangrene when it made its first appearance in a wound. They first applied nitric acid or another escharotic to the slough, which began working to disintegrate the infected tissue so that it would separate from the healthy tissue. Most surgeons used an anesthetic before they began working with the wound because of the severe pain caused by the acid. They had to apply the escharotic thoroughly to have a chance of halting the infection. Dr. W. W. Keen, a Union surgeon, explained his technique.

[The escharotic] must be unsparingly applied to every spot and surface involved. Stumps must be laid bare and apparently ruined; sinuses must be fully exposed, and the disease relentlessly pursued to its furthest refuge. . . . The work must be thorough and complete and the remedy applied everywhere—not only to the surfaces diseased, but also to those laid bare by the knife, and even somewhat to the sound parts beyond, or the disease will spread inevitably, and kindness well meant will be really unintentional cruelty. I generally used, as a means of application, a stick rather than a mop, since, if sharp pointed, it penetrates to places which will remain untouched if a mop is used.[126]

Keen's approach was correct. Since gangrene is an anaerobic organism (meaning that it thrives in the absence of oxygen) the debridement treatment must go beyond the infected tissue into the seemingly healthy tissue or the infection will spread and the symptoms will return.

After the debridement of the slough, the wound was washed thoroughly with soap and water, any dead parts were removed, and then a "disinfectant" was applied to the wound and around its edges. Labarraque's solution of chlorinated soda, tincture of iodine, turpentine, Dakin's solution, and bromine were all commonly used for this purpose. Although these disinfectants were not antibiotics (they did not directly kill the bacteria), they did help the patient by inhibiting the further growth of the microorganism by making its environment less favorable. Dry lint or lint soaked with turpentine was then placed over the wound. Finally, the wound was bandaged, and the patient ordered to rest. Sometimes a drip irrigation of a disinfectant solution or a poultice of various ingredients (including elm, charcoal, yeast, or carrots among others) was used to promote healing. Various deodorants were used as needed to help mask the offensive smell of the decaying tissue.[127] Surgeon Keen used permanganate of potash for this purpose.[128]

A critical feature of the treatment of such wounds was the isolation of gangrenous patients from those with wounds healing without any obvious complications. The isolation of infected patients was something that seems to have varied from hospital to hospital. Some facilities simply did not have the space or design to separate the infected patients from the rest of the group entirely. Instead, they would partially remove the patient by placing him behind a screen or put him at the far end of the ward. If a common cleaning pail or sponge was used to clean all the wounds in that ward, then that practice did practically nothing to halt the spread of the infection, which further confounded the doctors.

At Chimborazo and other large general hospitals, true isolation was more feasible. The surgeons at Chimborazo designated Ward A of each division to be set aside for serious cases of infection. Small Sibley tents were also erected to house the more contagious patients, to prevent the contamination of a large ward, which would then require thorough cleaning and whitewashing before any new patients could be admitted to it. At Winder Hospital, however, evidence exists of a lack of proper isolation of contagious infection. Surgeon-In-Chief A. G. Lane ordered the medical officer at Winder No. 2 "to send all cases of erysipelas, gangrene and pyaemia to the tents erected for that purpose upon the development of the first symptoms of either disease."[129] Evidently, the patients there were being isolated only after the advanced signs of the infections. Private T. M. Earnhart, admitted to Winder Hospital with a gunshot wound in June 1864, reported that he was assigned to a ward "full of gangrene and erysipelas, which were said to be highly communicable."[130]

Further isolation practices were adopted during the latter years of the war and some innovative practices attempted. Private Earnhart wrote, "Each patient had his own wash pan and sponge, which were intended to be used by no one else; but . . . it was up to me to keep a lookout that my pan and sponge were used on no one else and that no one else's were used on me."[131] Obviously, the connection had been made by medical officers between the cleansing of wounds and the spread of infection, but the implementation of the idea lacked enforcement.

Interestingly, if a modern physician were asked to treat a gangrenous wound with the medications and tools available to the Civil War surgeon, the treatment would change very little. The major difference would be to employ the antiseptic agents earlier, when the wound is first examined, instead of waiting until the infection is in full bloom.

Erysipelas, occurring less frequently than gangrene, was another infectious threat to wounded patients. The *Medical and Surgical History* described it as an "inflammation of the skin, originating from a wound, [which] quickly extended over the surrounding parts . . . accompanied by an exceedingly high fever."[132] The affected area usually began at the wound site, then spread into surrounding areas. The average duration of the ailment was eleven days, by which time the patient began to recover or had developed serious complications that overshadowed the erysipelas. Recurrent attacks were common. Union army records reveal a mortality rate of 41 percent for patients with erysipelas. However, many of these patients had also developed gangrene, haemorrhage, or pyaemia; only about 15 percent of the recorded fatal cases were directly attributed to erysipelas.[133]

Civil War physicians debated whether erysipelas was caused from the general environment or from a specific contagion, but all noticed that the infection generally occurred in crowded, badly ventilated rooms, in which it quickly spread. The most effective treatment was bromine, either applied topically as a solution or sprayed as a vapor throughout the ward. The most common treatment included immediate isolation and the free use of various disinfectants, such as iodine and creosote, applied topically.[134] At Chimborazo, one case of erysipelas of the face was treated with stimulants freely administered, whiskey, brandy, quinine, tonics, and cold dressings. After a few days, the patient became "decidedly better."[135]

Union surgeons M. Goldsmith and B. Woodward reported their success with bromine vapor to check the quick spread of the infection at the Park Barracks Hospital in Louisville: "[S]ince the use of bromine in vapor not one case originated in the crowded wards of the barracks, in which, before its use, from five to eight cases of erysipelas a week had occurred."[136] However, the news of the effectiveness of bromine evidently never reached most physicians, who did not use bromine to treat the infection.

The modern treatment for this bacterial infection includes penicillin or erythromycin for the infection and cold packs and aspirin for the pain. Today's physicians rarely have to worry about the serious complications of this infection, which are streptococcal gangrene and bacteremia.[137] Thus, this malady provides a good example of the great advantage that access to antibiotics gives to modern physicians. Even if Civil War doctors had understood this infection, they could have done nothing else for it.

In cases of both gangrene and erysipelas, Civil War surgeons did attempt to use topical and oral solutions to combat the infection. However, the effectiveness of these medications had to be weighed against their toxic effects. Mercury compounds exert antibacterial action but are highly toxic to tissues and penetrate poorly. A solution of carbolic acid (phenol) is an effective anti-infective drug against certain bacteria and fungi, but systemic toxicity limits its clinical usefulness.[138] The efforts to use any medications to combat the infections that the physicians did not understand was admirable but little likely to succeed. But again the trial-and-error approach was their only tool.

Another great infectious threat was pyaemia, a bacterial blood-poisioning.[139] Civil War surgeons also referred to this condition by the terms septaemia, septicaemia, ichorrhaemia, pyohaemia, and toxaemia, depending on the various symptoms and lesions it produced. The modern equivalents would be bacteremia and septic shock. The contraction of this infection resulted in almost certain death, regardless of the location of the wound infected initially or the medical treatment ordered. Civil War physicians usually prescribed a good diet and the use of tonics and stimulants. Approximately two-thirds of cases died within the first seven days of contracting this infection; very few survived longer than twenty days. According to Union statistics, of 2,818 cases only 17 patients recovered—a mortality rate of 97.4 percent.[140] In comparison, modern treatment includes transferring the patient to intensive care, administering oxygen, special antibiotics, and drugs to strengthen the heart and lessen inflammation; even today between 50 and 90 percent of cases are fatal.[141] Pember remembered it as the disease "from which no one ever recovers. . . . The only cases under my observation that survived were two Irishmen, and it was really so difficult to kill an Irishman that there was little cause for boasting on the part of the officiating surgeons."[142]

The fourth major example of serious infection was tetanus. Fortunately, this type of infection was not contagious. Although it struck only a small percentage of wounded patients—only .2 percent in the Union army—it received a great deal of attention from physicians because of its violence and quick progression. Of the 505 reported Union cases, 89.3 percent died.[143] The infection normally manifested itself within a few days of the injury. After the onset, the large majority of cases died within a week. Among the few tetanus patients who survived, the symptoms were treated and checked before the infection had time to develop fully. Civil War physicians were completely mystified by the cause of this ailment. Explanations included "excessive heat, exposure to cold and damp air, draughts, neglect of thorough and early cleaning of the wound channel, pressure of millies and bone splinters and of bandages on nerves, [and] injuries to nerves while searching for foreign bodies or while performing ligations and excisions."[144] One medical historian has concluded that the large outbreaks of tetanus, which were few, usually occurred "[i]n battles such as Antietam, where stables were used for hospitals."[145] The treatments varied extensively; the most popular remedies were chloroform, ether, opiates, and stimulants. Other recorded attempted treatments included oral doses of yellow jasmine, camphor, nitric acid, and castor oil, external applications of ice, electric currents, lime and opium poultices, and injections of opiates, tobacco, turpentine, vinegar, and brandy.[146]

Modern physicians realize that tetanus is an acute infectious disease caused by *Clostridium tetani*—anaerobic, spore-forming, gram-positive bacilli. The symptoms of stiffness, especially of the jaw, and severe muscle spasms are caused by a toxin that the bacillus emits. Prognosis is extremely poor if treatment of the infection is delayed, because the toxin cannot be neutralized once it is fixed in the nervous system.[147] If left untreated, the infection results in a very violent and painful death. For this reason, modern physicians encourage immunization against tetanus and immediately treat patients with deep puncture wounds with the immune globulin if any question exists about whether the patient has been immunized within the last five years. Careful wound debridement is also essential. If the immunization is not given and tetanus develops, even a moderate case can require intubation, gastric feeding tubes, oxygen, thorough wound debridement, pain medication, antibiotics, and drugs to manage muscle spasms, in addition to administering the antiserum.[148]

Besides the medical challenges brought about by horrible wounds and the constant threat of infection, Civil War surgeons also had to deal with other problems caused by the physical conditions of the battlefields and hospitals. The unclean conditions of most field and camp hospitals, where wounds were primarily dressed, severely hampered physicians' efforts to treat patients effectively. The presence of maggots in wounds was "frequently an annoying complication," prohibited only by cleaning and re-dressing the wound every few hours.[149] The common treatments for maggots were topical applications of oil of turpentine, petroleum, kerosene, or tobacco. Although the problem was not nearly as common in the larger general hospitals, the medical staffs had to deal with it when patients had been transferred in from a distance. As morbid as it sounds, maggots did actually help some patients by disposing of the dead tissue in the wounded area, although the patient suffering from a maggot infestation probably could see nothing positive about their presence.

Rats were another problem common to most hospitals. Although little good can be said about the rodents, at least one did help a patient at Chimborazo. Pember remembered the incident:

> A Virginian had been wounded in the very center of the instep of his left foot. The hole made was large, and the wound sloughed fearfully around a great lump of proud flesh which had formed in the center like an island. The surgeons feared to remove the mass, as it might be connected with the nerves of the foot, and lock-jaw might ensue. Poor Patterson would sit on his bed all day gazing at his lame foot and bathing it with a rueful face, which had brightened amazingly one morning when I paid him a visit. He exhibited it with great glee, the little island gone, and a deep hollow left, but the wound washed clean and looking healthy.
>
> Some skillful rat surgeon had done him this good service while in the search for luxuries, and he only knew that on awakening in the morning he had found the operation performed.[150]

Relating the stories of rats and maggots in hospitals helps us to remember the sorts of conditions under which Confederate physicians operated. Within that environment, the success that they achieved was remarkable. Not only were they working from a medical theory that today we would consider incorrect and using a variety of substitute medications, but they were also dealing with numerous problems that challenged their efforts to provide the healthy supportive conditions their patients needed for their bodies to heal. The physical and administrative situation at Chimborazo allowed physicians to devote more time trying to understand the medical challenges they faced and to adjust their treatments to provide the best care possible to their patients.

Many physicians who served in the Confederate or Union army were able to learn a great deal from their wartime experiences. The large numbers of patients they treated with similar medical problems prompted them to keep an open mind when determining diagnosis and treatment. Their access to fellow physicians and to medical journals allowed them to become aware of new or unfamiliar tools or treatments and to discuss the theories and questions that arose as they went about their daily rounds. They learned how to safely use anesthetic agents and other medications and how best to prevent and treat infectious disease. They developed surgical skills and the wisdom to know when to best apply those skills. They achieved a new level of confidence about their medical knowledge and related that confidence to their patients.

Interestingly, a review of cases of wounded in both the Confederate and Union armies reveals that America's physicians were dancing all around the germ-theory concept as they treated their patients, even though they continued to cling to the traditional ideas of contagion. They were unable to break completely with their old ideas, but their experiences with the vast numbers of patients they treated with similar problems prompted them to try different treatments that went beyond the logic of their existing medical theories. When the new treatments worked, as when they gave each wounded patient his own bucket and sponge for wound-cleaning, they adopted it—regardless of whether they felt they understood it. Through this commonsense, trial-and-error approach they made much medical progress in the right direction. As we have seen, often the physicians in Civil War hospitals had the right idea but lacked the understanding to implement the treatment earlier or more completely.

CHAPTER 7

The Closing

By the end of the war, much improvement had been achieved within the Confederate Medical Department. Thousands of medical officers and stewards had gained experience in the care and treatment of large numbers of sick and wounded in a hospital setting. One Confederate physician commented several years after the war that the doctor was "more practically efficient and useful, at the bedside now, than perhaps he has ever been before, and the whole country is now furnished with a medical corps which the war has thoroughly educated and reliably trained." Another Confederate doctor agreed: "I have lost much, but I have gained much, especially as a medical man. I return home a better surgeon, a better doctor."[1] Jefferson Davis stated, "The only department that was not demoralized was the Hospital Department that was well in hand and doing efficient service until the end of the war."[2]

Chimborazo Hospital and its sister institutions achieved much progress during the war, but by 1865 the situation of the Confederacy had become desperate and was growing worse every day. The lack of supplies reached critical levels, and the appeals of medical officers to Confederate agencies fell on deaf ears. Phoebe Pember explained the situation after February 1865: "Then came the packing up, quietly but surely, of the different departments. Requisitions on the medical purveyor were returned unfilled, and an order from the surgeon-general required that herbs instead of licensed medicines should be used in the hospitals."[3]

John Jackson, assigned as officer of the day at Chimborazo No. 2, wrote the following in his report dated January 13, 1865: "On examination I find scarcity of fuel as to an extent of discomfort and exposure of patients; office so uncomfortable that ordinary comfort is out of the question. There is also complaint of want of sufficient food—candles wanting for necessary purposes. P.S. In ward A—No wood for 2 days."[4] On March 7 E. S. Harrison reported "*no* wood, a scarcity of bed clothes in some wards & of chamber pots," and on March 19 he stated, "[T]he hospital is in by no means a comfortable condition, from scarcity of fuel and bed clothing. And the sick fairing badly for want of proper diet and medicines." On March 21 Harrison lamented, "not a sufficient number of attendants in some of the wards to keep them tolerably decent."[5]

Earlier that month, on March 14, Carrington wrote to McCaw, "[I]n future use all means at [your] disposal to secure by purchase or from the Commissary the necessary subsistence for patients and attendants."[6] Even at this point, McCaw continued to work to improve the condition of the food supplied to his patients; he requested an increase in the meat ration. Capt. F. F. Myer denied McCaw's request, explaining why in a letter to Major B. P. Nolan, the chief commissary of Virginia:

> On account of the great scarcity of meat I have been compelled to issue, in liew [*sic*] thereof, two glls of Molasses or 1/4 of a pound of Lard to attendants, and guards at hospitals, this course was actually necessary, and as soon as the emergency has passed the issue of 1/3 of a pound of bacon will be resumed. Surely, if men in the field submit to such deprivations these men ought. Compliance with the request of Surg McCaw will be increasing the ration of meat, and at this time it is impossible to issue them the present ration. It would, therefore, add to the embarrassments of the department, without, benefitting the hospitals.[7]

By the end of March, Medical Department officials were aware of the imminent surrender of Richmond. On March 21 Carrington wrote his final official letter to McCaw: "You are directed, without delay, to select for transfer to Hospitals in Danville, Farmville, or Lynchburg, all patients who will not be injured by transportation, and who will not be fit for duty within 15 days."[8]

By this time, the rate of exchange of Confederate money to specie was one hundred dollars to one dollar. The price of butter had risen to twenty dollars per pound. Historian Ernest Furgurson, reporting the observations of a Union spy in Richmond, wrote, "Because the government was snatching horses off the streets, suburban farmers were refusing to bring food to market, and 'people are really in a deplorable state. . . . We are in an awful situation.'"[9] Thomas Conolly, an Irish member of Parliament who had just arrived in Richmond, described the city as "wretched." "Shops were open with nothing to sell, strewn with empty packing boxes and straw. Streets were full of 'rowdies.'"[10]

The situation of the Confederate army was just as critical. General Sheridan was coming from the Shenandoah Valley and General Sherman from the south to join General Grant. According to Furgurson, when all Union troops arrived, "Grant would soon have roughly 280 [thousand] in the east. To deal with them, the Confederates had about 65 [thousand]."[11] To help supplement the severe shortage of manpower, a very hesitant Confederate Congress finally responded to Lee's call for black troops by passing the bill on March 13. Nine days later the first three companies of enlisted black soldiers paraded in Richmond's Capitol Square. "Two companies," Furgurson noted, "were made up of attendants and nurses from Winder and Jackson hospitals, the third from Captain Turner's recruiting station. The hospital companies were not picked men but of 'all sizes, from three feet to six foot six.'"[12] It was too late to matter. President Jefferson Davis sent his wife and family south to Florida. On March 29 the Union army's final campaign began.

To defend against Union raiders, all of the attendants and remaining patients in Richmond's hospitals had been assigned to standby battalions. As Furgurson stated, "Stacks of rifles, ammunition, and equipment waited between wards. At Chimborazo, H. E. Wood, a wounded sergeant of the Eighteenth Virginia, organized clerks, stewards, and convalescents. He stated, "Scarcely an able-bodied soldier among them. I suppose every State in the Southern Confederacy was represented.'"[13]

On Sunday, April 2, the War Department received the news that Grant had broken through the defenses around Petersburg and was on his way to Richmond. Confederate officials immediately began burning their records. By midnight no Confederate or Virginia state official remained in Richmond. The army left the city as well. That same evening, Major Isaac H. Carrington followed orders and set a fire to destroy the cotton, tobacco, and other commodities left in the city's warehouses; the fire soon got out of control. Union troops advancing on Richmond met the city's officials, who surrendered the city at 6:30 A.M. on April 3.[14]

All day Sunday Pember watched the evacuation from her view at Chimborazo. She recalled:

> Then I walked through my wards and found them comparatively empty. Every man who could crawl had tried to escape a Northern prison. Beds in which paralyzed, rheumatic, and helpless patients had laid for months were empty. . . . Those who were compelled to remain were almost wild at being left. . . . I gave all the comfort I could, and with some difficulty their supper also, for my detailed nurses had gone with General Lee's army, and my black cooks had deserted me.[15]

The next day, she watched the long columns of Union soldiers. "She was impressed by the Yankees' quietness and courtesy, and the fat horses and shiny trappings that contrasted so much with the wasted appearance of the departed Confederates," Furgurson wrote of Pember's reaction.[16]

Monday brought the surrender and occupation of Chimborazo Hospital. Years later, McCaw related the event to a newspaper reporter:

[Maj. Gen. Godfrey Weitzel] rode up the hill and through the post;
he was received by our whole corps of officers in full uniform.
Dr. Alexander Mott was chief medical officer on the staff of General
Weitzel, and as the staff rode into the post, he exclaimed: "Ain't that
old Jim McCaw"? I said "Yes! and don't you want a drink?" He said,
Yes, and the General will take one, too, if you will ask him!" And it
goes without saying that the invitation was duly extended and accepted
con amere. Mott said the General wants to do anything at all for you
which you may want him to do. I asked for a general permit for passage
out of the lines for myself and for all of my officers, which was promptly
granted. As a proof of the good feeling which always existed from the
beginning to the very end of the war, General Godfrey . . . took [the
commandant and his entire medical corps] under his protection, and
issued a verbal order that all Confederate soldiers there should be taken
care of under all circumstances. Gen. Weitzel further offered to put the
commandant in the general service of the United States, so that he
might issue requisitions, etc. and have the same filled as any other
medical director in the U.S.A. But I respectfully declined the proffered
appointment, as General Lee had not then surrendered, and I was still
in the service of the C.S.A., but voluntarily continued to perform all the
duties incident to the position I held, and never solicited anything at
all from them other than the passes in and out of the lines.[17]

That morning three Union surgeons inspected Chimborazo's wards, accompanied by the appropriate surgeons-in-charge. Soon after, one of the hospital's divisions was cleared out so that it could house Union patients. Pember stated, "[T]heir patients laid by the side of our own sick so that we shared with them, as my own commissary stores were still well supplied."[18] On Thursday, Chimborazo and all other Richmond hospitals were ordered to transfer their remaining patients to Jackson Hospital. At Chimborazo, Pember "protested bitterly against this, as they were not in a fit state for removal, so they remained unmolested."[19]

Over the next week or so, Pember continued her work at Chimborazo, defiantly challenging anyone who threatened her authority to do so. Before Union guards arrived at the hospital, she had to confront a group of "hospital rats" who broke into her quarters to steal the thirty gallons of whiskey located there. She quickly recognized the men and questioned the ringleader, whom she described as "an old enemy, who had stored up many a grievance against me." She told him, "Wilson . . . you have been in this hospital a long time. Do you think from what you know of me that the whiskey can be taken without my consent?" He grew very angry and insolent, grabbed Pember by her shoulder, and "called [her] a name that a decent woman seldom hears and even a wicked one resents." She responded by pulling out her "little friend," which she cocked, then ordered them to leave, stating, "for if *one* bullet is lost, there are five more ready, and the room is too small for even a woman to miss six times." They grudgingly left. Pember then reinforced her position by nailing the lid from a flour barrel across the door. That night she slept by the whiskey barrel with a candle, some matches, and her pistol within reach.[20]

Another challenge was to continue to provide food for her patients. When Pember learned that the Union soldiers had confiscated her hospital's supplies, she immediately dressed in her best clothing, then "walked into Dr. M's office, now Federal headquarters . . . [and] accosted the principle [sic] figure seated there, with a stern and warlike demand for food, and curt inquiry whether it was their intention to starve their captured sick."[21] The officer in charge gave her permission to drive her ambulance into Richmond to obtain food. She left with a bag of coffee and a demijohn of whiskey and returned with a live calf that provided beef for her patients.

A short time later, this time needing sugar, Pember went to her hospital's commissary. "Two Federal guards were in charge, but they simply stared with astonishment as I put aside their bayonets and unlocked the door of the place with my pass-key, filled my basket, with an explanation to them that I could be arrested whenever wanted at my quarters." From that point until she left Chimborazo a few weeks later the guards left her alone. "No explanation was ever given to me why I was allowed to come and go, nurse my men and feed them with all I could take or steal." An errand boy later reported to her that a Union sutler had confidentially told him that the U.S. surgeon-in-charge was "awful afraid of her."[22] When her patients were finally transferred to Jackson Hospital, she accompanied them. She remained there "till all the sick were either convalescent or dead."[23]

Very soon after Chimborazo's patients were transferred, the wards of the hospital began being used for a very different purpose. On June 3, 1865, M. Jennie Armstrong reported in a letter to Rev. William George Hawkins that an afternoon school for the newly freed slaves had been opened at Chimborazo that week. When it opened, 180 students, "young and old," attended the school. By November 1 attendance had increased to 345 pupils: 166 males and 179 females. Twenty-six students were under six years old, 26 were older than sixteen, and the rest fell in the middle. Six teachers from New England taught the students, using six of Chimborazo's wards. The school's headmaster was Mr. J. Walker, a graduate of Amherst

College. Rev. R. M. Manley, who was a chaplain and an officer of the Freedmen's Bureau, was also usually in attendance. By October 23 a night school of approximately 200 students had also been organized at the facility. Of those attending the school, teacher Jennie Armstrong reported, "The children, although laboring under many disadvantages, conduct themselves with remarkable propriety. I have yet to see the evidence of willful disobedience. In comprehending the first steps of knowledge, they give evidence of clear minds, acute powers of observation, and excellent memories." Later in the letter she wrote, "The quiet, steady perseverance of these people in spite of all obstacles in the past, is a strong guarantee for the future."[24]

The Chimborazo school, described in letters published in *The National Freedman* as a "mission field," also helped freed blacks by providing some clothing and food to the most destitute. One letter explained, "A systematic course of visitation was early commenced by the teachers among the people, which has revealed many scenes of utter destitution that are painful to witness."[25] The following example is typical of the letter's content: "An aged woman was found in a dark cabin without fire, literally clothed in rags. She had eaten nothing but a few cabbage leaves for two days. While clothing her from our scanty supply of garments, a bag of dry beans were [sic] found, and given to her, she clutched them with her long bony fingers, exclaiming: 'God bless you, this is the best of all.'"[26]

The clothing at Chimborazo school came from aid societies in the North, which also sent cloth, boots, shoes, and some cash. According to the headmaster, "The clothing and cloths are given to the necessitous, and sold at a very small price to those able to pay."[27] The school's teachers determined the amount of charity given based on personal examinations of the individual cases who requested help. Charitable items were given not only to those who came to Chimborazo but also to the truly destitute in the area. The money received from the sale of clothing was spent mainly on fuel, although some went for food to the sick or hungry.[28] On February 1, 1866, Miss I. G. Campbell, one of the teachers at Chimborazo, wrote, "The supply of clothing, which, when it first arrived, seemed almost inexhaustible, is nearly gone; at least the warm garments."[29] Besides requesting more clothing, Campbell also asked for secondhand bed quilts or army blankets. Evidently, the appeals of Maney and Campbell worked. According to the May 1866 issue of the paper, a total of $850 in cash, in addition to more clothing and shoes, was received by the Chimborazo school between February 1 and April 14.[30]

In addition to providing education, clothing, and food, the Chimborazo facility had by early 1866 become a refugee camp. Its buildings, described by the school's headmaster as being of the "shabbiest construction," housed over fifteen hundred newly freed slaves, most of whom were women, children, or elderly individuals with no place to go.[31]

Evidently, the school and refugee camp lasted only a short time. In 1870 seven acres of Chimborazo Hill was purchased by Joseph Bacher, a Prussian immigrant who had earlier developed prosperous breweries in Vermont and Pennsylvania. Bacher and his family came to the Richmond area to pursue the promise of prosperity in postwar Virginia. Bacher used a series of underground cellars that had been constructed on the hill by two previous beer makers to store his beer. After only a few years, Bacher's business failed; he found that the cellars had not been dug deeply enough, making the temperatures in the cellars too high for the beer to keep. Bacher had not understood how difficult it would be for him to obtain ice in the area. He moved back to Vermont, selling the land to the city of Richmond.[32]

In 1874 the city of Richmond purchased the site of Chimborazo Hospital in order to use it as a park. The area became more accessible to the Richmond public in 1897 when the Richmond Traction Company extended its "splendid transportation facilities."[33] Apparently the site never caught on, since the city temporarily turned possession of the plateau over to the U.S. government so that it could be used as a United States Weather Bureau station, which it was from 1909 to 1954. On May 26, 1934, a bronze tablet was placed atop a waterworn boulder on the edge of Chimborazo Hill to memorialize the hospital and its success. In mid-1941 Richmond City Councilman Emmett Perkinson proposed using the old beer storage cellars at Chimborazo as air-raid shelters; the idea died after an examination of the unstable condition of the cellars.[34] In 1959 the National Park Service occupied the old Weather Bureau building and designated the area as the Richmond National Battlefield Park.[35]

Although Chimborazo's direct influence in the world of medicine stopped when it was closed at the end of the Civil War, the impact of those responsible for organizing and running the facility lasted many more years. Moore remained in Richmond after the war. Because he had sufficient means, he did not maintain an active practice. "By 1875 he was fully retired from clinical practice and devoted his attention to the development of education and agriculture in the South. . . . Moore was especially interested in measures used to improve the health of both school children and teachers," noted Ira Rutkow.[36] Corresponding to his interests, Moore served from 1874 to 1881 as a member of the Executive Board of the Virginia Agricultural Society and from 1877 to 1889 as a member of the Richmond City School Board. When the Association of Medical Officers of the Confederate States formed in 1874, Moore was elected as its president. Moore died in Richmond on May 31, 1889, and was buried at Hollywood Cemetery.[37]

After all her patients left Jackson Hospital, Phoebe Pember found herself with only "a box full of Confederate money and a silver ten-cent piece" to show for her four years of work at Chimborazo. She spent the dime on a box of matches and five cocoa-nut [sic] cakes. To explain her purchase, she stated, "Should any one ever be in a strange country where the currency of which he is possessed is valueless, and ten cents be his only available funds, perhaps he may be able to judge of the difficulty of expending it with judgment."[38] After staying in Richmond a short time, living off of the kindness and generosity of friends there, Pember returned to Georgia. She wrote the memoirs of her experiences at Chimborazo sometime between 1865 and 1879, when they were first published. "She apparently wrote from memory though she probably had at hand some papers and documents bearing on her war-time experience," Bell Irvin Wiley speculated.[39] Until she died on March 4, 1913, she spent a great deal of time traveling, both in the United States and abroad.

McCaw returned to life as a civilian doctor. He resumed his medical practice and continued his teaching at the Medical College of Virginia. In 1869 he shifted his teaching interests and became professor of the theory and practice of medicine, a position he held until 1884. He also served as chairman of the medical faculty from 1868 to 1871 and then as dean of faculty from 1871 to 1883. In 1882 the governor of Virginia attempted to increase his influence over the school by appointing an entirely new Board of Visitors. Acting under Governor Cameron's instructions, the board assembled at the medical college to organize and inspect the books. Its efforts were stopped by Drs. McCaw and J. S. Wellford, another faculty representative. McCaw had called in enough police to prevent the board members' entrance to the facility. The police supported McCaw over the governor. When the case went before the Virginia Supreme Court, the court ruled in favor of McCaw; the original Board of Visitors was reinstated.[40] After leaving his position as dean, McCaw served on the Board of Visitors and then finally as chair of the Board of Visitors until his retirement.

Throughout the rest of his life he continued to exhibit his dedication to patient care and medical knowledge. In August 1869 he chaired a special committee of the Richmond Academy of Medicine that produced a report on the best way to combat the influences of malaria. In November 1870 he presided over a meeting of 147 physicians to reorganize the Medical Society of Virginia, of which he became president. In 1871 he contributed an article to the *Virginia Clinical Record*. In 1874 he was one of three physicians whom the Association of Medical Officers of the Confederate Army and Navy requested to prepare a sketch of the organization and services of the Confederate Medical Department. He served as the president of the Richmond Academy of Medicine, on the Board of Directors of the Pinel Hospital (designed especially for mentally ill patients), as a consultant for Richmond's Eye, Ear, and Throat Infirmary and Dispensary, and as a volunteer physician for the Sheltering Army Hospital.[41]

McCaw did not retire from active practice until 1901, when he was honored with a rare banquet by Richmond's Academy of Medicine for his fifty-seven years of contributions to the medical community. The guest list bridged the gap between academia and medicine, rural and urban practitioners, and revealed the widespread admiration felt for McCaw. Despite all of his achievements, it is notable that

McCaw always considered Chimborazo Hospital as his greatest accomplishment.[42] Upon his death, on August 13, 1906, at the age of eighty three, his obituary appeared in the *British Medical Journal*, a rare honor for an American physician. The notice stated, "Dr. McCaw was a typical Virginia gentleman of the old school, devoted to the highest interests of his native city and State, and few practitioners have been so universally beloved in their community as he."[43]

Today, nothing remains of the "Hospital on the Hill" except for its legacy. Part of the flat plateau on which it stood is a grassy park that surrounds the Richmond Battlefield Park visitors center. The rest has been developed into residential neighborhoods. Attempts to examine life in the hospital's wards are complicated by the lack of a complete set of records. When Richmond fell and most of the hospital's patients and staff left the facility, most physicians took their case books with them, wanting to preserve as much of their research as possible. The remainder of Chimborazo's records stayed at the hospital until requested by the U.S. Army Surgeon General's Office when it began compiling information for *The Medical and Surgical History of the War of the Rebellion*.[44] The records were eventually turned over to the National Archives for safekeeping.

Along the way and through the years, much of the information has been lost. One hundred and twenty-three bound volumes of Chimborazo's records can be found today. Unfortunately, since Richmond burned, very few of the corresponding records from the Confederate Medical Department survived to help fill the gaps. However, a thorough examination of the records that remain, when placed within the context on other information on the Civil War and medical practice during the nineteenth century, allows an evaluation of the impact of Chimborazo Hospital on medicine in general.

CHAPTER 8

An Evaluation

Chimborazo Hospital treated almost eighty thousand patients during its four years of operation. We have examined its facilities, its organization, its staff, and the medical treatment of its patients. With this information in hand, we may ask just how good was Chimborazo Hospital? I propose that we judge the hospital by five criteria: its quality of organization, its quality of patient care, its level of innovation, its compliance with military regulations, and its perceived success or failure as seen through the eyes of those who lived and worked there.

The quality of organization appears to have been very high at Chimborazo. McCaw's development of the multi-hospital Chimborazo post quickly became a model for the establishment of other large hospitals. The division surgeons had the authority to run their divisions and supervise their staffs without having to worry about the issues of the post. The presence of the matrons served as a check against problems that would hurt the welfare of the patients. McCaw's good communication with his division surgeons and matrons, as well as his frequent walks through the hospital's wards, enabled the organizational structure to work well. The stability of leadership by McCaw, the division surgeons, and the division matrons also contributed to the smooth operation of the facility. The fact that the hospital's administration listened to and acted on patient complaints also speaks well of the organization.

The medical treatment received by patients at Chimborazo was as good or better than at any other hospital during the Civil War. The easiest way to measure the quality of medical care is to look at mortality rates. Early statistics provided by reports from the hospital show the mortality rate to be around 6 percent. After the war, on various occasions, Chimborazo's surgeons reported the number to be approximately 9 percent. The best statistical report, which evaluated the hospital's records from 1861 to 1865, puts the mortality rate at 11.39 percent. The average mortality rate for Union hospitals was 10 percent. The difference could have very easily been from the lack of supplies in the last year of the war.

Another way to evaluate medical care is to look at the treatment given to patients. A comparison of Chimborazo's records and medical cases reported in the multivolume *Medical and Surgical History of the Civil War* reveal that the methods of treatment were similar. It is notable that Chimborazo performed and reported on many of the new treatments tried at other major military hospitals. Innovations in patient care, such as separating patients by ailment, and the performance of clinical drug trials does suggest that Chimborazo Hospital either initiated or quickly adopted many new techniques that saved patients' lives.

Chimborazo was innovative from its very beginning. Its construction was of the "pavilion" style, making it the first American hospital, North or South, to be built in this new way, which was designed for maximum ventilation. Its organization as a grouping of hospitals placed under a surgeon-in-chief and designated an independent army post gave McCaw much more authority than a hospital's surgeon would have had under another arrangement. The creative use of the hospital fund was another innovation—one that allowed for the procurement of critical supplies and healthy foods when such was scarce. With regard to medical care, Chimborazo's surgeons kept up with recent medical advances, applied that knowledge to the treatment of their patients, and kept careful personal journals in which to report the results. Even more telling, perhaps, is the spirit of some of Chimborazo's records; the staff seems to have a readiness to take advantage of opportunity and a willingness to try new things.

Compliance with military regulations was one area where Chimborazo's performance suffered. This deficiency was probably due in large part to McCaw's personality. Moore wrote to McCaw many times in the early years of the war to inform him that things at Chimborazo were not being done through proper channels or according to military regulations. McCaw administered his hospital from his authority, checked initially only by his own dedication to patient care. He tended to act on an issue and then wait on Moore to tell him whether he had the authority to do it. As the administrator of a large military hospital, this approach caused problems. The innovation of McCaw, as discussed above, can be viewed as a positive feature of the hospital. However, innovation in bureaucratic matters does not fit well into a military organization.

Since medical treatment is such a highly personalized activity, the perception of Chimborazo is also important. As seen through the comments of patients noted at the end of chapter 4, many patients were pleased with the treatment they received at Chimborazo. Although the hospital environment was far from perfect, most patients understood that the hospital's staff members were doing all they could to help them recover. The positive accounts by patients are even more impressive when compared to the common antebellum negative perception of hospitals.

In her memoirs, Phoebe Pember took pride in her time at Chimborazo. Her account included many of the ugly details of hospital life, but the tone of her writing indicates a deep satisfaction with her abilities as a matron. She knew that she had made a positive difference in the lives of the men who lived in her wards. McCaw and other surgeons at Chimborazo also remembered their experiences fondly. Despite his numerous achievements after the Chimborazo years, McCaw always considered the hospital as his greatest accomplishment.

The other question that must be asked is how Chimborazo Hospital compared to other Civil War hospitals, Union and Confederate. Chimborazo had some unique advantages that allowed it to excel in ways other Confederate hospitals could not. Its healthy location, its stability of location, and its proximity to Richmond allowed the facility to develop its procedures and to try innovative medical treatments that could not have been done easily at a hospital that had to move frequently. Its proximity to Richmond allowed for easy access to medical experts and to the senior staff of the Confederate Medical Department. Unfortunately, its closeness to the city also caused enormous supply challenges that could not be easily overcome by the end of the war. As a Confederate hospital, it did not have the benefits of supplies or staff that the United States Sanitary Commission provided to similar hospitals in the North. However, its administration was not confronted with the political struggles that faced the leadership of Union hospitals and the Union Medical Department.

In the final analysis, both Union and Confederate hospitals made remarkable strides during the war. Surgeons faced enormous challenges as the war began. As Alfred Jay Bollet wrote, "With no models to draw on, both sides' Medical Departments devised extensive workable hospital systems."[1] Medical officers constructed hospitals with designs consistent with the latest medical thought; developed an efficient ambulance system; learned to work with (and around) quartermasters for their patients' food, clothing, and medicines; trained nurses to care for patients; and developed specialty hospitals. While accomplishing their administrative tasks, they worked to practice medicine in a thoughtful manner that would maximize any new knowledge that might be gained from the large number of patients they treated. When the war ended, these doctors returned to their homes and their medical practices with a greater understanding of medicine and an awareness of the possibilities for successful medical treatment in an institutional setting.

NOTE ON SOURCES

T his work began in graduate school as I was researching general information on Civil War hospitals and came across a reference to Chimborazo Hospital in a footnote. The records of most Richmond hospitals were burned in the Richmond fire, which was set as the Confederate government evacuated the city in 1865 in the face of the advancing Union army. Most other sources I had seen regretted that no records were available for Richmond hospitals. However, this obscure footnote reported that, contrary to popular belief, the records of Chimborazo Hospital were housed at the National Archives in Washington, D.C. A quick call to the archivist there one afternoon between classes verified that the records were indeed available to review. My dissertation topic was born.

My husband and I traveled to Washington, D.C., the next summer and found 123 volumes of Chimborazo records plus 66 other volumes of related Confederate hospital or medical department records. Since Chimborazo Hospital was located outside the city, it did not destroy its records. After the war ended, the boxes and volumes of information were put together with other miscellaneous Confederate government records that had survived and sent to Washington. The compilers of the *Medical and Surgical History of the War of the Rebellion* did review Chimborazo's records as they compiled their information on the hospital. They used a complete patient register (probably the one from Chimborazo's main administrative office) to compile their statistics of patient admissions, disease classification, and mortality. Since then, the main register has been lost. It is not part of the current collection at the National Archives. Without it, there is no opportunity to do a more thorough statistical analysis of patients or mortality rates, so I have relied on the *Medical and Surgical History* for that information.

Among the most valuable of Chimborazo's volumes were sets of orders and memorandums sent between James Brown McCaw, the surgeon-in-chief at Chimborazo, and his staff. These volumes gave me a great deal of insight into the personality and management style of McCaw and the relationship he had with his staff. Also valuable were volumes of orders and memos sent between McCaw and either Surgeon General Samuel Preston Moore or Medical Director William Carrington. Interesting logistical facts were discovered in volumes containing information on hospital purchases, personnel registers, records from the bakery, and reports by the officer of the day for one division. A few volumes with prescription information and accounts of specific medical cases was valuable for its reporting of common practices as well as unexpected results. Many of Chimborazo's volumes were patient registers of various sorts. Some register volumes appeared to be sections of the main register, but most were division registers. Several of the register volumes were duplicates. Quite a few volumes contained records on coarse paper that had become illegible because of the age and character of the paper and ink. Unfortunately, the collection of Chimborazo's records is not complete. I have done my best to ensure that the significant features of the hospital's records are adequately reported here, since few people have the time or opportunity to view the documents for themselves.

The other sixty-six related volumes provided more information on the Confederate medical system and its hospitals. Six volumes survived from Winder hospital (Chimborazo's sister hospital in Richmond). Several of these volumes were also patient or personnel registers, but some of the information adds to the understanding of large Confederate hospitals. Unfortunately, no other information on Winder survives to my knowledge, thus limiting one's ability to compare and contrast the two sister mega-hospitals in Confederate Richmond. It does appear from the records that Winder's overall patient numbers were slightly greater than Chimborazo's, even though Winder did not open until 1862. However, Chimborazo still rightfully maintains its distinction as the largest Confederate hospital, because its average daily census remained consistently higher than Winder's.

With regard to medical treatment, the most important primary sources other than Chimborazo's records were the *Confederate States Medical and Surgical Journal* and the *Medical and Surgical History of the Civil War*. These collections gave insight into the common medical treatments as well as the more innovative treatments. Also valuable to my understanding of the medical concepts was Thomas Watson's *Lectures on the Principles and Practice of Physic* (an 1858 medical textbook), current medical and anatomy books, and the ability of my husband (a pharmacist) to explain things to me.

The most important primary source that put a human face on the picture of Chimborazo Hospital was the memoirs of Phoebe Yates Pember, who served as a matron at the hospital. She kept a journal of her experiences during the war and then used it to compile her memoirs after the war. I will be forever grateful for her desire to preserve her experiences at Chimborazo. She published her initial memoir in 1879, but it has gone through many editions and reprints since then. There are a few times when I quote Pember from H. H. Cunningham's *Doctors in Gray*. The quotations that Cunningham reports are not in the memoirs as currently published. Since Cunningham did not provide notes or a bibliography in his work, it is entirely possible that he found those quotations in other works that were available at the time. I used these quotations after considering their consistent nature and the reputation of Cunningham's book.

NOTES

PREFACE

1. Mary C. Gillett, *The Army Medical Department, 1818–1865* (Washington, D.C.: United States Army Center of Military History, 1987), 117. In comparison, the rate at the U.S. Army hospital at Vera Cruz during the Mexican War was approximately 12 percent and the rate at the New Orleans Charity Hospital approximately 15 percent.
2. Charles E. Rosenberg, *The Care of Strangers: The Rise of America's Hospital System* (Baltimore: Johns Hopkins Univ. Press, 1987), 93.
3. Richard Boies Stark, "Surgeons and Surgical Care of the Confederate States Army," *Virginia Medical Monthly* 88 (Oct. 1961): 604.
4. Alfred Jay Bollet, *Civil War Medicine: Challenges and Triumphs* (Tucson, Ariz.: Galen, 2002), 444.

CHAPTER 1

1. John Duffy, *From Humors to Medical Science: A History of American Medicine,* 2nd ed. (Urbana: Univ. of Illinois Press, 1993), 153.
2. Duffy, *From Humors to Medical Science,* 153.
3. Bonnie Ellen Blustein, *Preserve Your Love for Science: The Life of William A. Hammond, American Neurologist* (New York: Cambridge Univ. Press, 1991), 7, 53–65; Charles J. Stille, *The History of the United States Sanitary Commission: The General Report of Its Work During the War of the Rebellion* (Philadelphia: J. B. Lippincott, 1866), 63. Frederick Law Olmsted, appointed to serve as the chief executive officer of the USSC, stated that the object of the USSC was "to *supplement* Government deficiencies . . . [and] to endeavor to secure from every Government official the full measure of his responsibility" (Stille, *History of the United States Sanitary Commission,* 77; emphasis in original). Also important, the USSC's recommendation of William Hammond for surgeon general was probably the deciding factor for his appointment.
4. Duffy, *From Humors to Medical Science,* 158.
5. A good example of the high turnover rate among hospital administrators occurred at Lincoln Hospital, a model Union hospital located near Washington, D.C. When Lincoln admitted its first patients in December 1862, Henry Bryant was the surgeon-in-charge. G. S. Palmer replaced Bryant in July 1863. Roberts Bartholow succeeded Palmer. According to Gloria R. Irby, "It is possible that Bartholow's appointment was political; it corresponds directly with the removal of Hammond [as surgeon general]." Finally, from March 1864 until August 1865, Cooper McKee served as the surgeon-in-charge. See Irby, "Chimborazo and Lincoln Hospitals" (master's thesis, Humboldt State College, 1967), 56.
6. H. H. Cunningham, *Doctors in Gray: The Confederate Medical Service,* 2nd ed. (Baton Rouge: Louisiana State Univ. Press, 1960), 21.
7. Stark, "Surgeons and Surgical Care," 604–5.

8. Samuel Preston Moore's Confederate Army Service Record, Record Group 109, National Archives, Washington D.C. Many secondary sources give the date of his appointment as July 30, 1861.

9. Wyndham B. Blanton, *Medicine in Virginia in the Nineteenth Century* (Richmond, Va.: Garrett & Massie, 1933), 277.

10. Rutkow, "Samuel Preston Moore," vi–viii.

11. James M. McPherson, *Ordeal by Fire: The Civil War and Reconstruction* (New York: Alfred A. Knopf, 1982), 206–7.

12. Cunningham, *Doctors in Gray*, 27.

13. Pyre Porcher, "Samuel Preston Moore," *Southern Historical Society Papers* 33 (1893): 114–15.

14. Cunningham, *Doctors in Gray*, 31. The officer's name was not provided.

15. J. Boulware, assistant surgeon, Sixth South Carolina Volunteers, July 24, 1862, qtd. in Robert E. Denney, *Civil War Medicine: Care and Comfort of the Wounded* (New York: Sterling Publishing Co., 1994), 135.

16. Clifford Dowdey, *Experiment in Rebellion* (Garden City, N.Y.: Doubleday, 1946), 241.

17. Cunningham, *Doctors in Gray*, 165.

18. Cunningham, *Doctors in Gray*, 166.

19. Mary Boykin Chesnut, *Mary Chesnut's Civil War*, ed. C. Vann Woodward (New Haven, Conn.: Yale Univ. Press, 1981), 81.

20. Blanton, *Medicine in Virginia*, 212–22; Robert W. Waitt, *Confederate Military Hospitals in Richmond*, Official Publication No. 22, Richmond Civil War Centennial Committee (Richmond, Va.: City of Richmond, 1964), 5, 8–9; Dowdey, *Experiment in Rebellion*, 240. These hospitals continued to provide care for Richmond's civilians during the war.

21. Blanton, *Medicine in Virginia*, 300–301. The Catholic sisters referred to were the Cornette Sisters from Emmitsburg, Maryland, who had been asked by Dr. Gibson to help the sick and wounded in Richmond. Most of the sisters of this order served at the St. Anne's Military Hospital during the war. See Denney, *Civil War Medicine*, 24.

22. Cunningham, *Doctors in Gray*, 45.

23. Cunningham, *Doctors in Gray*, 28.

24. James Brown McCaw, qtd. in "Of Chimborazo Park," clipping dated Aug. 11, 1897, from an unidentified Richmond newspaper; copy in Chimborazo File, Richmond National Battlefield Park Headquarters, Richmond, Va.

25. Mary Newton Stanard, *Richmond: Its People and Its Story* (Philadelphia: J. P. Lippincott Co., 1923), 171.

26. "Beer, Not Wine, First Stored in Chimborazo Park Cellars," clipping dated July 3, 1941, from an unidentified Richmond newspaper; copy in Chimborazo File, Richmond National Battlefield Park Headquarters.

27. Dowdey, *Experiment in Rebellion*, 303–4.

28. John R. Gildersleeve, "History of Chimborazo Hospital, Richmond, Va., and Its Medical Officers During 1861–1865," *Virginia Medical Monthly* 88 (Oct. 1961): 588.

29. Medical Purveyor's Office to McCaw, Oct. 15, 1861, Records of Chimborazo Hospital, Record Group 109, War Department Collection of Confederate Records, National Archives, Washington, D.C., vol. 707: 1. Hereafter, this collection of materials will be referred to as Chimborazo Records, followed by the relevant volume and page numbers.

30. Adj & Insp Gen Office, special order 198, Nov. 31, 1861, Chimborazo Records, vol. 707: 3.

31. McCaw, qtd. in "Of Chimborazo Park."

32. *Richmond Whig,* Nov. 1, 1861.

33. Nathan Rosenberg, "America's Rise to Leadership," in *America's Wooden Age: Aspects of its Early Technology,* ed. Brooke Hindle (Tarrytown, N.Y.: Sleepy Hollow Restorations, 1975), 44.

34. Samuel Stout, qtd. in "Chimborazo Hospital," unpublished report, Chimborazo File, Richmond National Battlefield Park Headquarters, 25.

35. Robert Bruegmann, "Architecture of the Hospital: 1770–1870, Design and Technology" (Ph.D. diss., Univ. of Pennsylvania, 1976), 19–21, 108–9. The Nightingale quotation appears on page 109 of this dissertation.

36. Bruegmann, "Architecture," 113.

37. Charles S. Tripler, qtd. in Cunningham, *Doctors in Gray,* 50.

38. Russell V. Bowers, "A Confederate General Hospital: Chimborazo Post (1862–1865)," *The Scarab,* Nov. 1962, 2.

39. James H. Brewer, *The Confederate Negro: Virginia's Craftsmen and Military Laborers, 1861–1865* (Durham, N.C.: Duke Univ. Press, 1969), 96; Moore to McCaw, Jan. 29, 1862, Chimborazo Records, vol. 707: 33.

40. "Chimborazo Hospital," *Richmond Whig,* Nov. 1, 1861.

41. Moore to McCaw, Dec. 5, 1861, Chimborazo Records, vol. 707: 16.

42. Moore to McCaw, Mar. 18, 1862, Chimborazo Records, vol. 707: 51.

43. To McCaw, Mar. 31, 1862, Chimborazo Records, vol. 707: 59.

44. Moore to McCaw, Apr. 2, 1862, Chimborazo Records, vol. 707: 122, 125b.

45. Moore to McCaw, Apr. 21, 1862, Chimborazo Records, vol. 707: 79.

46. Waitt, *Confederate Military Hospitals,* 11–12.

47. Moore to McCaw, Apr. 25, 1862, Chimborazo Records, vol. 707: 81.

48. Denney, *Civil War Medicine,* 97; Alexander Lane, "Address to the Association of Army and Navy Surgeons of the Confederacy," *Southern Practitioner* 26 (1904): 34–41; Charles F. Ballou, "Hospital Medicine in Richmond, Virginia During the Civil War: A Study of Hospital No. 21, Howard's Grove, and Winder Hospitals" (master's thesis, Virginia Polytechnic Institute and State University, 1992), 25–29. Winder Hospital was named after General John Henry Winder, who served as the provost marshal in Richmond throughout the war.

49. Cullen, *Richmond Battlefields,* 9.

50. Cullen, *Richmond Battlefields,* 25.

51. The surgeons-in-chief of Howard's Grove Hospital, in order of their service, were Dr. James Bolton, Dr. T. P. Temple, and Dr. P. M. Palmer. The hospital eventually had a capacity of approximately eighteen hundred patients, cared for by eighty-five employees. Its sixty-two buildings included a laundry, bakery, storehouses, and recreational facilities. Waitt, *Confederate Military Hospitals,* 20.

52. John B. Jones, July 3, 1862, qtd. in Denney, *Civil War Medicine,* 129.

53. Mrs. Sally Putnam, July 3, 1862, qtd. in Denney, *Civil War Medicine,* 130.

54. Moore to Carrington, Feb. 2, 1863, Surgeon General's Office Records, Record Group 109, War Department Collection of Confederate Records, National Archives, Washington, D.C., vol. 740: 67.

55. Cunningham, *Doctors in Gray,* 50; Waitt, *Confederate Military Hospitals,* 9.

56. Waitt, *Confederate Military Hospitals,* 20. Jackson Hospital was named in honor of General Thomas J. "Stonewall" Jackson.

57. Howard's Grove Hospital Records, 1862–63, Record Group 109, War Department Collection of Confederate Records, National Archives, Washington, D.C., vol. 192. This collection of materials will hereafter be referred to as Howard's Grove Records.

58. Moore to McCaw, Mar. 18, 1862, Chimborazo Records, vol. 707: 51.
59. Carrington to McCaw, July 24, 1863, Chimborazo Records, vol. 708: 174.
60. Blustein, *Preserve Your Love for Science,* 7, 63–65.

CHAPTER 2

1. *Regulations for the Army,* 239–40; Glenna R. Schroeder-Lein, *Confederate Hospitals on the Move: Samuel H. Stout and the Army of Tennessee* (Columbia: Univ. of South Carolina Press, 1994), 111.
2. *The Richmond Examiner,* n.d., copy in Chimborazo file, Richmond National Battlefield Park Headquarters, Richmond, Va. The support staff included the men who worked in the commissary and the quartermaster's office at Chimborazo and the hospital's other supply agents.
3. Dowdey, *Experiment in Rebellion,* 303. Dowdey also stated, "[H]is appointment was one of those happy choices that occasionally in wartime produce results far beyond the immediate requirements."
4. James Brown McCaw was born in Richmond on July 12, 1823. His grandfather, Dr. James Drew McCaw, came to Virginia in 1771. His father, Dr. William R. McCaw, graduated from Edinburgh. Samuel Mordecai, *Richmond in By-Gone Days* (1860; rpt. Richmond, Va.: Dietz Press, 1940), n.p.
5. Valentine Mott (1785–1865) had taught at the medical schools of Columbia and Rutgers before he assisted in establishing the medical department at the University of the City of New York, where he taught surgery and surgical anatomy. As a surgeon he gained worldwide recognition for being the first to perform several surgical procedures successfully, including surgeries for aneurisms and an amputation at the hip joint. His surgical record included almost 1,000 amputations, 150 operations for bladder stones, and 40 ligations of large arteries. His reputation continued to grow as he became an authority on surgical anesthesia after its introduction in 1846. "Valentine Mott," *Dictionary of American Biography,* ed. Dumas Malone, vol. 7 (New York: Charles Scribner's Sons, 1933), 290.
6. Blustein, *Preserve Your Love for Science,* 4. Blustein discusses two professors who probably made the biggest impact on her subject, Dr. William Hammond. McCaw would have also had these professors. One was Martyn Paine, the professor of the "institutes of medicine and materia medica." As Blustein wrote, "Paine touched on the ways in which the 'effects of life' could be modified 'by the mind itself'" (4). The other was John William Draper, an eminent scientist, who served as the professor of chemistry at the medical school. Blustein reports that Draper "tried earnestly to convey the excitement of the age to his students. 'There is hardly a book of science that comes across the Ocean which does not bring with it new facts, the coordination of which with those that are known, remains to be made,' Draper lectured. 'The formative process is beginning; a few years will give us a science, which will bring more revolutions in medicine, than that changeable science has even yet witnessed.' . . . Draper made a special point of demonstrating experiments in such a way as to make them repeatable by the students themselves in the expensive new laboratory" (5).
7. The couple had nine children; two of his sons became physicians and one of his daughters married a physician. His son Walter Drew McCaw rose to the rank of

brigadier-general and served as the chief surgeon in the American Expeditionary Forces in World War I. The daughter married Dr. Christopher Tompkins; their son also became a physician, serving Richmond as a skilled doctor and a professor at the medical college. The Tompkins-McCaw Library at the Medical College of Virginia is named in honor of this dedicated medical family. This information about McCaw's family is drawn from various materials, including the following: W. T. Thompson Jr. and E. Randolph, "Man of the Hour," *The Scarab*, Nov. 1962, 6, 21; Cunningham, *Doctors in Gray*, 51 n; and an obituary for McCaw in *The British Medical Journal* 2 (1906): 601.

8. Thompson and Trice, "The Man of the Hour," 6.
9. *Stethoscope* 4 (1854): 770, qtd. in Blanton, *Medicine in Virginia*, 119.
10. Blanton, *Medicine in Virginia*, 116–17.
11. "James Brown McCaw," in *Dictionary of American Biography*, ed. Dumas Malone (New York: Charles Scribner's Sons, 1933), 575–76.
12. "James Brown McCaw," 576. Another source stated, "Dr. James B. McCaw was a Virginia gentleman of the highest type, of commanding figure, courteous to all and generously endowed by nature with the most attractive qualities of body and mind" (Thompson and Trice, "Man of the Hour," 6).
13. Phoebe Yates Pember, *A Southern Woman's Story: Life in Confederate Richmond, 1862–1865*, ed. Bell Irvin Wiley (Marietta, Ga.: Mockingbird Books, 1992), 16–17.
14. Ernest B. Furgurson, *Ashes of Glory: Richmond at War* (New York: Alfred A. Knopf, 1996), 153.
15. Schroeder-Lein, *Confederate Hospitals on the Move*, 17–21.
16. Blanton, *Medicine in Virginia*, 117; Blustein, *Preserve Your Love for Science*, 3.
17. Blustein, *Preserve Your Love for Science*, 54.
18. Blustein, *Preserve Your Love for Science*, 7, 56 (quotation).
19. Blustein, *Preserve Your Love for Science*, 63.
20. Blustein, *Preserve Your Love for Science*, 231, 5–7, 12, 63–75.
21. Blustein, *Preserve Your Love for Science*, 7–8. Hammond was forced out of the surgeon general position because of a political scandal initiated by Secretary of War Edwin Stanton, a major opponent of Hammond.
22. Moore to McCaw, Dec. 30, 1861, Chimborazo Records, vol. 707: 23.
23. Schroeder-Lein, *Confederate Hospitals on the Move*, 58.
24. Dowdey, *Experiment in Rebellion*, 305.
25. Cunningham, *Doctors in Gray*, 75.
26. A. S. Mason, chief surgeon's office, to McCaw, order, Dec. 7, 1862, Chimborazo Records, vol. 707: 26.
27. To McCaw, July 18, 1862, Chimborazo Records, vol. 707: 141; To McCaw, July 27, 1862, Chimborazo Records, vol. 707: 147.
28. N. J. Walker to McCaw, Oct. 3, 1863, Chimborazo Records, vol. 708: 232.
29. Pember, *Southern Woman's Story*, 36.
30. A. S. Mason, chief surgeon's office, to McCaw, Feb. 13, 1863, Chimborazo Records, vol. 708: 48.
31. Pember, *Southern Woman's Story*, 57.
32. B. H. Huestis, sergeant commander of the guard, to McCaw, Nov. 10, 1864, Chimborazo Records, vol. 709: 226. No reply was found in the records.
33. I. N. Fauit to McCaw, July 22, 1864, Chimborazo Records, vol. 709: 154.
34. Pember, *Southern Woman's Story*, 45.

35. *Regulations for the Army,* 193.
36. Schroeder-Lein, *Confederate Hospitals on the Move,* 73.
37. W. J. Coffur, surgeon-in-charge of receiving hospital, to McCaw, Nov. 13, 1862, Chimborazo Records, vol. 707: 207.
38. Chimborazo Records, n.d., vol. 709: 344.
39. General Benjamin W. S. Cabell to McCaw, Apr. 3, 1862, Chimborazo Records, vol. 707: 64–56.
40. McCaw to Cabell, Apr. 5, 1862, Chimborazo Records, vol. 707: 66.
41. McCaw to William Clopton, n.d., Chimborazo Records, vol. 708: 43.
42. F. W. Bridgeforth to Dr. E. W. Johns, forwarded to Dr. James McCaw, Aug. 1, 1862, Chimborazo Records, vol. 707: 156.
43. E. E. Coerall to McCaw, n.d., Chimborazo Records, vol. 709: 171.75.
44. Coerall to McCaw, Chimborazo Records, vol. 709: 171.75.
45. Colonel Joel R. Griffin, Eighth Georgia, Petersburg, Virginia, to McCaw, Nov. 12, 1864, Chimborazo Records, vol. 709: 227.
46. Carrington to McCaw, Mar. 3, 1864, Chimborazo Records, vol. 709, 47. The nature and duties of the Executive Committee are unknown. In this letter, Carrington informed McCaw of a meeting of the group at his house on March 4 at 6:00 P.M. He stated, "Several Matters of importance require immediate decision."
47. Confederate Service Records of P. F. Browne, William A. Davis, Stephen E. Habersham, E. M. Seabrook, and Edwin H. Smith, Record Group 109, National Archives, Washington, D.C. Browne helped organize Winder Hospital and the general hospital at Danville, Virginia. Davis helped organize the general hospital at Harrisburg, Virginia, served for a brief period in the Army of Northern Virginia, and served in the Reserve Surgical Corps. Seabrook also served with the Reserve Surgical Corps. Smith served a short time at Texas Hospital in Richmond.
48. Surgeon General's Office, circular no. 1, Nov. 23, 1861, Chimborazo Records, vol. 408: 1.
49. Pember, *Southern Woman's Story,* 18.
50. McCaw to Chimborazo No. 2, n.d., Chimborazo Records, vol. 408: 6.
51. Some outstanding physicians were given the rank of surgeons even though they were recent medical school graduates or had not yet practiced medicine for five years. See Schroeder-Lein, *Confederate Hospitals on the Move,* 70.
52. Schroeder-Lein, *Confederate Hospitals on the Move,* 70; Chimborazo Records, vol. 88: 625.
53. Chimborazo Records, vol. 88: 625.
54. *Regulations for the Army,* 241.
55. Surgeon General's Office to McCaw, circular, Mar. 24, 1863, Chimborazo Records, vol. 740: 159.
56. Carrington to McCaw, May 15, 1864, Chimborazo Records, vol. 709: 99.
57. P. F. Browne, surgeon-in-charge, Chimborazo No. 1, to McCaw, June 18, 1863, Chimborazo Records, vol. 708: 160.
58. Carrington to McCaw, June 19, 1863, Chimborazo Records, vol. 708: 160b.
59. S. E. Habersham, surgeon-in-charge, Chimborazo No. 2, general order, Dec. 14, 1861, Chimborazo Records, vol. 408: 4.
60. Surgeon W. A. Davis to McCaw, Feb. 1, 1864, Chimborazo Records, vol. 317: 86.
61. Surgeon R. S. Peebles, Medical Director's Office, to Surgeon Seabrook, Chimborazo, Apr. 20, 1864, Chimborazo Records, vol. 709: 85.

62. S. E. Habersham, surgeon-in-charge, Chimborazo No. 2, to assistant surgeons, n.d., Chimborazo Records, vol. 408: 29.

63. Officer of the Day Report, Dec. 8, 1864, Chimborazo Records, vol. 324: n.p.

64. Moore to Chimborazo's assistant surgeons, order, Chimborazo Records, vol. 25; Mar. 1862, Chimborazo Records, vol. 707: 55.

65. The assistant surgeons at Chimborazo to Moore, n.d., Chimborazo Records, vol. 97: n.p.

66. E. W. Gordon to S. E. Habersham, report of the officer of the day, Nov. 15, 1864, Chimborazo Records, vol. 324: n.p.

67. Kaufman, *Homeopathy in America,* 23; see also Joseph F. Kett, *The Formation of the American Medical Profession: The Role of Institutions, 1780–1860* (New Haven, Conn.: Yale Univ. Press, 1968), 29–31. In this climate of limited medical education and licensure, numerous "irregular" medical sects, such as eclectics, Thomsonians, and homeopaths, had begun to challenge the ideas and treatments of "regular" or allopathic medicine. The success of regular physicians during the Civil War weakened much of the momentum of these alternative groups.

68. Cunningham, *Doctors in Gray,* 263.

69. Cunningham, *Doctors in Gray,* 257.

70. Cunningham, *Doctors in Gray,* 255.

71. Duffy, *From Humors to Medical Science,* 58.

72. *Regulations of the Army,* 242.

73. John Harley Warner, "The Fall and Rise of Professional Mystery," in *The Laboratory Revolution in Medicine,* ed. Andrew Cunningham and Perry Williams (New York: Cambridge Univ. Press, 1992), 128.

74. George B. Wood, qtd. in Gert H. Brieger, "Classics and Character: Medicine and Gentility," *Bulletin of the History of Medicine* 65 (Jan. 1991): 96–97.

75. Brieger, "Classics and Character," 94.

76. Surgeon General's Office, circular, Nov. 20, 1862, Chimborazo Records, vol. 546: 81.

77. Schroeder-Lein, *Confederate Hospitals on the Move,* 70. Schroeder-Lein's information came from reviewing samples of numerous examinations in Samuel Stout's records, now housed at the University of Texas.

78. *Regulations of the Army,* 242. Although regulations stipulated that an assistant surgeon had to serve for a minimum of five years before eligible for promotion to surgeon, the service records of many medical officers indicate that promotions of this nature were made throughout the war.

79. George E. Waller, letter, Twenty-fourth Virginia, qtd. in Cunningham, *Doctors in Gray,* 34–35. Arthur E. Peticolas was a member of the medical examining board who began teaching anatomy at the Medical College of Virginia in 1849 and was promoted to professor of anatomy in 1855. Peticolas was also a charter member of the Medical Society of Virginia and a contributor to the *Maryland and Virginia Medical Journal.* During the war, while continuing to teach, he served as a surgeon in a Richmond hospital. See Blanton, *Medicine in Virginia,* 47, 51, 55, 59, 91, 119, 413.

80. Schroeder-Lein, *Confederate Hospitals on the Move,* 70.

81. Surgeon General's Office to medical directors, circular, Dec. 15, 1863, Chimborazo Records, vol. 7: n.p.

82. Samuel Stout to T. G. Richardson, Mar. 28, 1864, qtd. in Schroeder-Lein, *Confederate Hospitals on the Move,* 92.

83. Moore to William Carrington, Sept. 23, 1864, Surgeon General's Office Records, vol. 741: 75.
84. Moore to Carrington, Mar. 1, 1864, Surgeon General's Office Records, vol. 741: 97.
85. Carrington to McCaw, 7 Febrary 1863, Chimborazo Records, vol. 708: 41.
86. Samuel Stout to Ferdinand E. Daniel, Sept. 21, 1898, qtd. in Schroeder-Lein, *Confederate Hospitals on the Move*, 78.
87. Schroeder-Lein, *Confederate Hospitals on the Move*, 80.
88. Pember, *Southern Woman's Story*, 57.
89. Pember, *Southern Woman's Story*, 26.
90. Pember, *Southern Woman's Story*, 57.
91. Chimborazo Records, vol. 440: 53, 55, 57. The physician's name was not listed. His case book recorded daily progress reports. In his initial entries he included such information as the patient's name, age, rank, occupation, regiment, state, company, brigade, date of wound, date of operation, anesthetic used, when last vaccinated (which was always filled in), kind of scar, result, and ward. He was obviously making an attempt to keep careful records but unfortunately was not entirely consistent with his information. The two surviving patients were S. N. Dawson, shot in his left ankle, and A. J. Compton, shot in both thighs. The third patient's name was not legible; he had been wounded in the right knee. The men had been wounded on February 6 and admitted to Chimborazo on February 9. In all three cases the wounds were treated with cold-water dressings, poultices, and Dover powder at night for pain. By February 18 the patients were transferred by Davis to Ward F. Various wounded patients from Wards B, C, M, and S were sent to Ward F. By April 1 Dawson and Compton had improved; the third patient developed pyaemia.
92. Pember, *Southern Woman's Story*, 18.

CHAPTER 3

1. Sister Mary Denis Maher, *To Bind Up the Wounds: Catholic Sister Nurses in the U.S. Civil War* (New York: Greenwood, 1989), 51.
2. Edmund Burke Haywood to Surgeon General Moore, qtd. in H.H. Cunningham, *Doctors in Gray*, 77.
3. R. L. Madison to Thomas Williams, Oct. 1861, Chimborazo Records, n.d., vol. 54: 15.
4. "An Act," Aug. 21, 1861, General Hospitals at Orange Court House and Farmville Records, Record Group 109, War Department Collection of Confederate Records, National Archives, vol. 546: 10; Moore to Thomas Williams, medical director of Virginia, forwarded to Surgeon R. L. Madison, Orange Court House Hospital, Nov. 14, 1861, Orange Court House and Farmville Records, vol. 546: 20.
5. Moore to Thomas Williams, forwarded to Surgeon R. L. Madison, Orange Court House Hospital, Nov. 14, 1861, Orange Court House and Farmville Records, vol. 546: 20.
6. "Regulations of General Hospital Camp Winder," *Confederate Imprints,* Collection of the Boston Athanaeum, Boston, Mass., 1063.
7. Brewer, *Confederate Negro*, 97–98.
8. McCaw to Carrington, Aug. 27, 1864, Chimborazo Records, vol. 709: 176.
9. Carrington to McCaw, Aug. 10, 1864, Chimborazo Records, vol. 709: 166; Carrington to McCaw, July 5, 1864, Chimborazo Records, vol. 709: 142.
10. T. N. Waul, "Special Report of the Committee appointed to examine into

Quartermaster's, Commissary & Medical Departments," Jan. 29, 1862, U.S. War Department, *War of the Rebellion: A Compilation of the Official Records of the Union and Confederate Armies* (Washington, D.C.: Government Printing Office, 1880–91), series 4, vol. 1: 883. This source will hereafter be referred to as *Official Records* and followed by series, volume, and page numbers.

11. T. N. Waul, "Special Report," qtd. in Cunningham, *Doctors in Gray*, 73.
12. Cunningham, *Doctors in Gray*, 73.
13. Kate Cumming, *Kate: The Journal of a Confederate Nurse*, ed. Richard Barksdale Harwell (Baton Rouge: Louisiana State Univ. Press, 1959), 38.
14. Pember, *Southern Woman's Story*, 105.
15. Cunningham, *Doctors in Gray*, 76.
16. Carrington, circular, June 5, 1863, Chimborazo Records, vol. 72: 2.
17. Cunningham, *Doctors in Gray*, 76.
18. Maurice Duke and Daniel P. Jordan, eds., *A Richmond Reader, 1733–1983* (Chapel Hill: Univ. of North Carolina Press, 1983), 107. Actually, according to Ernest B. Furgurson (*Ashes of Glory*, 4, 18), the figure is 37.6 percent. Of the remaining Richmonders, approximately one-third were white and the remaining third were foreign born, mainly Irish and German.
19. Furgurson, *Ashes of Glory*, 4.
20. Furgurson, *Ashes of Glory*, 20–21, 18.
21. Furgurson, *Ashes of Glory*, 19.
22. Furgurson, *Ashes of Glory*, 172.
23. McCaw to Moore, May 17, 1862, Chimborazo Records, vol. 707: 101.
24. Moore to McCaw, May 17, 1862, Chimborazo Records, vol. 707: 101.
25. Furgurson, *Ashes of Glory*, 172, 69.
26. Chimborazo Records, vol. 75.
27. Moore to Thomas Williams, medical director, forwarded to Surgeon R. L. Madison, Nov. 14, 1861, *Orange Court House and Farmville Records*, vol. 546: 20.
28. Chimborazo Records, vol. 98; Moore to McCaw, Mar. 18, 1863, Chimborazo Records, vol. 740: 147.
29. McCaw to Mrs. Harwood, Jan. 5, 1864, Chimborazo Records, vol. 709: 2.
30. Brewer, *Confederate Negro*, 98–99.
31. Brewer, *Confederate Negro*, 99. In 1863, slave owners received sixty thousand dollars from Chimborazo.
32. C. W. M. Hubball to McCaw, Dec. 6, 1862, Chimborazo Records, vol. 707: 223.
33. Brewer, *Confederate Negro*, 99.
34. Brewer, *Confederate Negro*, 101.
35. Colonel J. F. Gilmen, chief of Engineering Bureau, McCaw, Mar. 6, 1863, Chimborazo Records, vol. 708: 65; Carrington, circular, Aug. 24, 1863, Winder Records, Record Group 109, War Department Collection of Confederate Records, National Archives, Washington, D.C., vol. 547: 97.
36. Brewer, *Confederate Negro*, 101.
37. Carrington to McCaw, Dec. 27, 1864, Chimborazo Records, vol. 709: 254.
38. From an act passed by the Confederate Congress, Sept. 1862, quoted in Cunningham, *Doctors in Gray*, 76
39. Pember, *Southern Woman's Story*, 15.
40. William Alex Thorn to McCaw, Dec. 15, 1862, Chimborazo Records, vol. 707: 234. No response survives, but Goodwin was not found in Chimborazo's records.

41. Pember, *Southern Woman's Story,* 17.
42. Chimborazo Records, vol. 98, and vol. 322: 25. The wages paid to the matrons did increase during the war. In 1864 the matrons at Chimborazo received $250 per month for their services. See Pember, *Southern Woman's Story,* 134.
43. Morning report, Mar. 18, 1863, Chimborazo Records, vol. 322: 25.
44. "Regulations of General Hospital Camp Winder," *Confederate Imprints,* 1063. The "ladies' kitchen" was the kitchen that cooked the food for the hospital's invalid patients; all those patients who could walk took their meals in the division's convalescent dining room, run by the steward.
45. "Duties of the Chief Matron of Laundry Department," Okmulgee Confederate Hospital, Georgia, *Confederate Imprints,* 1033.
46. Pember, *Southern Woman's Story,* 16.
47. Pember to Eugenia Phillips (her sister), Nov. 29, 1862, in Pember, *Southern Woman's Story,* 112.
48. Pember, *Southern Woman's Story,* 19.
49. Pember, *Southern Woman's Story,* 19–20.
50. Pember, *Southern Woman's Story,* 22.
51. Pember, *Southern Woman's Story,* 23.
52. Pember, *Southern Woman's Story,* 20.
53. Pember, *Southern Woman's Story,* 23.
54. Pember, *Southern Woman's Story,* 60.
55. Pember, *Southern Woman's Story,* 24.
56. Cunningham, *Doctors in Gray,* 73.
57. Pember, *Southern Woman's Story,* 5.
58. Pember, *Southern Woman's Story,* 24.
59. Pember, *Southern Woman's Story,* 51.
60. Pember, *Southern Woman's Story,* 52. Pember added, "The reply [to her note] would be the same silly question I so often had to meet: 'Did Mrs. —— [*sic*] consider herself a lady when she wrote such notes?' 'No,' was always the indignant answer."
61. Pember, *Southern Woman's Story,* 51.
62. Pember, *Southern Woman's Story,* 32.
63. Pember, *Southern Woman's Story,* 33.
64. Pember, *Southern Woman's Story,* 33.
65. Pember, *Southern Woman's Story,* 35.
66. Pember, *Southern Woman's Story,* 35.
67. Carrington to McCaw, Apr. 11, 1863, Chimborazo Records, vol. 708: 99.
68. S. E. Habersham to McCaw, Chimborazo Records, n.d., vol. 708: 102.
69. Pember, *Southern Woman's Story,* 36.
70. Pember to Phillips, Sept. 9, 1863, in Pember, *Southern Woman's Story,* 120.
71. Pember, *Southern Woman's Story,* 138
72. Pember, *Southern Woman's Story,* 38. Miss G. probably refers to Miss Katie Ball, who was Pember's most trusted assistant matron.
73. Pember, *Southern Woman's Story,* 57.
74. Denney, *Civil War Medicine,* 303.
75. Pember, *Southern Woman's Story,* 88.
76. Pember, *Southern Woman's Story,* 88.
77. Pember, *Southern Woman's Story,* 52.

78. Pember, *Southern Woman's Story,* 46.

79. Cunningham, *Doctors in Gray,* 85.

80. Pember, *Southern Woman's Story,* 29.

81. Pember, *Southern Woman's Story,* 29.

82. Pember to Phillips, Jan. 30, 1863, in Pember, *Southern Woman's Story,* 115.

83. Pember, *Southern Woman's Story,* 78.

84. Pember, *Southern Woman's Story,* 90.

85. Pember, *Southern Woman's Story,* 89.

86. Pember to Lou Gilmer of Savannah, Dec. 30, 1863, in Pember, *Southern Woman's Story,* 129.

87. Pember, *Southern Woman's Story,* 78. When Pember was unable to find an escort to accompany her back to Chimborazo, "general advice was unanimously given to 'go alone,' on the grounds that women had become entirely independent at this time" (Pember, *Southern Woman's Story,* 79).

88. Moore to McCaw, Mar. 5, 1863, Chimborazo Records, vol. 708: 61. No other information about this incident is in the records; McCaw's response was not recorded.

89. Gillett, *Army Medical Department, 1818–1865,* 130, 156.

90. Gregory J. Higby, *In Service to American Pharmacy: The Professional Life of William Procter, Jr.* (Tuscaloosa, Ala.: Univ. of Alabama Press, 1992), 10.

91. Higby, *In Service to American Pharmacy,* 14–15.

92. Cunningham, *Doctors in Gray,* 75.

93. A correspondent named W. C. Warren asked McCaw find a place at Chimborazo for "a young gentleman of great worth" who "has been Steward in this Hospital for many months." He "was a student of Medicine before hostilities commenced— He wishes to be transferred to Richmond, that he may attend the Med. Lectures during the coming winter" (Warren to McCaw, Aug. 24, 1863, Chimborazo Records, vol. 708: 205). Another man, George W. Trice, also wrote to ask for a job as steward at Chimborazo: "When I saw you in June last you promised if I would write to you before the session of the Medical College commenced you would try and make some arrangement so that I could attend" (Trice to McCaw, Sept. 1, 1863, Chimborazo Records, vol. 708, 209).

94. Carrington to McCaw, Nov. 4, 1864, Chimborazo Records, vol. 709: 219.

95. McCaw to Carrington, Sept. 9, 1863, Chimborazo Records, vol. 708: 216.

96. "Regulations of General Hospital Camp Winder," *Confederate Imprints,* 1063.

97. Pember, *Southern Woman's Story,* 35.

98. Carrington to McCaw, May 22, 1864, Chimborazo Records, vol. 709: 107.

99. Schroeder-Lein, *Confederate Hospitals on the Move,* 74.

100. Carrington to Virginia Hospitals, Sept. 3, 1863, and Moore to Medical Directors, circular, Aug. 27, 1863, Medical Director's Office Records, Record Group 109, War Department Collection of Confederate Records, vol. 557: n.p. The three surgeons on this examining board were C. I. Clark, O. A. Crenshaw, and O. F. Marson; Marson was replaced on September 11 by T. M. Palmer.

101. Instructions to the board of examiners, n.d., Medical Director's Office Records, vol. 557: n.p.

102. McCaw to Carrington, Sept. 9, 1863, Chimborazo Records, vol. 708: 216.

103. Examination Board Report, n.d., Medical Director Office Records, vol. 557: n.p. Smith was one of the older stewards, at thirty-five years old. Most stewards were in their twenties.

CHAPTER 4

1. Letter to Mary A. Livermore, qtd. in Mary A. Livermore, *My Story of the War: A Woman's Narrative of Four Years of Personal Experience* (Hartford, Conn.: A. D. Worthington Co., 1889), 126–27.
2. Blanton, *Medicine in Virginia*, 301.
3. Samuel Stout, "Some Facts of the History of the Organization of the Medical Service of the Confederate Armies and Hospitals," *Southern Practitioner* (Jan 1903), 29, qtd. in Schroeder-Lein, *Confederate Hospitals on the Move*, 48.
4. Rosenberg, *Care of Strangers*, 98.
5. Nicholas A. Davis, *The Campaign from Texas to Maryland with the Battle of Fredericksburg* (1863; rpt. Austin, Tex.: Steck Co, 1961), 68.
6. Pember, *A Southern Woman's Story*, 43.
7. Pember, *Southern Woman's Story*, 43–44.
8. In the first years of the war the baggage checks were simply pieces of cardboard with numbers on them. New printed baggage check forms were adopted as of July 6, 1863, for use throughout the Confederate Medical Department. See McCaw to Carrington, Aug. 3, 1863, Chimborazo Records, vol. 708: 187.
9. *Regulations for the Army*, 10.
10. 1863, Chimborazo Records, vol. 708: 47.
11. Pember, *Southern Woman's Story*, 37–38.
12. McCaw, order, Dec. 2, 1861, Chimborazo Records, vol. 408: 2. These orders marked Tuesday, December 3, as the first day that convalescent patients were to be fed three meals per day. In the winter, breakfast was served at 8:00 A.M., dinner at 2:00 P.M., and supper at 5:00 P.M.
13. Pember, *Southern Woman's Story*, 24.
14. McCaw, order, Dec. 2, 1861, Chimborazo Records, vol. 408: 2; punctuation added.
15. Pember, *Southern Woman's Story*, 24.
16. McCaw, order, Dec. 2, 1861, Chimborazo Records, vol. 408: 2; Pember, *Southern Woman's Story*, 22.
17. "Time Table of the Hours at which Medicines are to be given—For the guidance of Nurses, Matrons, & Wardmasters," Chimborazo Records, vol. 18: n.p. "Daily" and "AM & PM" times were 10:00 A.M. and bedtime.
18. Moore, circular, July 6, 1863, Confederate Medical Department Records, Record Group 109, War Department Collection of Confederate Records, National Archives, Washington, D.C., vol. 547: 77.
19. Pember, *Southern Woman's Story*, 28.
20. Pember, *Southern Woman's Story*, 18.
21. W. A. Davis to Carrington, Dec. 31, 1863, Chimborazo Records, vol. 317: 65.
22. S. E. Habersham to Brigadier General John M. Winder, n.d., Chimborazo Records, vol. 408, 4. Although this letter was not dated, it was found in a bound volume between items dated Dec. 14, 1861, and Jan. 23, 1862. "Hospital rats" were not only found at Chimborazo but at hospitals throughout the South. Matron Fannie Beers, who served at hospitals in the deep South, described the hospital rat in this way: "'[One] who at the first rumor of an approaching battle, had experienced 'a powerful misery' at the place where a brave heart should have been, and, flying to the rear, doubled up with rheumatism and out-groaning all the victims of *real* sickness or horrible wounds, had remained huddled up in bed until danger was over'" (Beers, qtd. in Schroeder-Lein, *Confederate Hospitals on the Move*, 116).

23. After December 1862 General Hospital No. 10, under the command of Medical Director William A. Carrington, was the designated officers' hospital. The facility had been the Union Hotel before the war. Chimborazo served as an overflow facility, according to a circular dated Dec. 4, 1862, from E. S. Gaillard (Chimborazo Records, vol. 408: 1). General Hospital No. 4, a Baptist girls' school before the war, was under the command of Dr. James P. Read; it began receiving officers for treatment in January 1863. Each facility had a capacity of over three hundred patients. See Waitt, *Confederate Military Hospitals in Richmond,* 11–13.
24. Pember to Mrs. Lou Gilmer, Apr. 15, 1864, in Pember, *Southern Woman's Story,* 143.
25. Carrington to General John H. Winder, Mar. 23, 1864, *Official Records,* series 2, vol. 6: 1084.
26. Carrington to General John H. Winder, Mar. 23, 1864, *Official Records,* series 2, vol. 6: 1085.
27. Carrington to McCaw, Apr. 30, 1864, Chimborazo Records, vol. 709, 89; McCaw to Carrington, May 12, 1864, Chimborazo Records, vol. 709: 98b.
28. Davis to McCaw, Mar. 14, 1862, Chimborazo Records, vol. 707: 46.
29. Surgeon L. Guild, inspector of hospitals, to McCaw, Mar. 15, 1862, Chimborazo Records, vol. 707: 47. On December 26, 1864, the Surgeon General's office issued a circular expanding this practice. This notice (Surgeon General's office to medical directors in the field and of hospitals, circular no. 13, Dec. 26, 1864, *Confederate Imprints,* 1000), stated, "The employment of negroes as teamsters and laborers, in the place of enlisted men, renders it necessary to provide special hospital accommodations for them." It ordered medical directors to reserve as many hospital tents or buildings as necessary to accommodate these patients.
30. Circular no. 13, *Confederate Imprints,* 1000
31. Patient Register, Sept. 1, 1864, Chimborazo Records, vol. 79: n.p.
32. W. A. Davis to McCaw, Jan. 19, 1864, Chimborazo Records, vol. 317: 81.
33. Pember, *Southern Woman's Story,* 67. According to Dr. Charles Cook, this was the only recorded birth in a Confederate hospital ("Chimborazo Hospital: Flagship Medical Center of the Confederacy" [presentation at the National Museum of Civil War Medicine, Frederick, Md., Aug. 1995]).
34. Davis, *Campaign from Texas to Maryland,* 128.
35. "Regulations of General Hospital Camp Winder," *Confederate Imprints,* 1063; "Regulations, Academy Hospital," *Confederate Imprints,* 1064; "Regulations, General Hospital Farmville," Orange Court House and Farmville Hospital Records, vol. 546: 145.
36. Schroeder-Lein, *Confederate Hospitals on the Move,* 46.
37. Assistant Inspector General to McCaw, n.d., Chimborazo Records, vol. 707: 149.
38. I. B. Yarrington to Carrington, Feb. 24, 1864, Chimborazo Records, vol. 709, 40. Yarrington was fifty-five years old in 1864.
39. Moore, circular no. 22, Dec. 3, 1864, Chimborazo Records, vol. 7: 9.
40. McCaw to Carrington, May 15, 1864, Chimborazo Records, vol. 9: 11.
41. McCaw to Carrington, Aug. 27, 1864, Chimborazo Records, vol. 709: 176. McCaw was also asking for more men to serve as nurses as well. Carrington replied, "Application has been made for several hundred conscripts to be sent to Richmond Hospitals. All available men that report will be sent to Chimborazo Hos."
42. Carrington to McCaw, Jan. 30, 1864, Chimborazo Records, vol. 709, 19. The names of the convalescents remained on the hospital's registers and are in their respective divisions. See McCaw, order, Feb. 15, 1864, Chimborazo Records, vol. 709: 22.

43. Adjutant attorney general to Carrington, Dec. 30, 1863, Chimborazo Records, vol. 708: 277.

44. Cunningham, *Doctors in Gray*, 92. It is not known whether Chimborazo had a library or provided newspapers to its patients.

45. Moore to McCaw, Oct. 9, 1863, Chimborazo Records, vol. 708: 236.

46. "Of Chimborazo Park."

47. Pember, *Southern Woman's Story*, 133.

48. Pember to Mrs. Lou Gilmer, Dec. 30, 1863, in Pember, *Southern Woman's Story*, 133; see also Pember, *Southern Woman's Story*, 87. This feat was particularly amazing when the prices of those items are considered. Mary Boykin Chestnut (*Mary Chesnut's Civil War*, 434) reported the cost of turkeys that winter as thirty dollars each.

49. Pember, *Southern Woman's Story*, 87.

50. Pember, *Southern Woman's Story*, 74.

51. Pember, *Southern Woman's Story*, 74. At that point Pember states that Confederate paper was worth sixty cents to the Union dollar.

52. McCaw to medical director, Oct. 11, 1862, Chimborazo Records, vol. 707: 185.

53. Moore to McCaw, Sept. 22, 1863, Chimborazo Records, vol. 708: 225.

54. Pember, *Southern Woman's Story*, 75.

55. *Richmond Daily Whig*, July 7, 1864.

56. Pember, *Southern Woman's Story*, 45.

57. Pember, *Southern Woman's Story*, 61.

58. Pember, *Southern Woman's Story*, 61.

59. Cunningham, *Doctors in Gray*, 85.

60. Pember, *Southern Woman's Story*, 65.

61. The smuggling of food and liquor to patients by visitors was a common problem. Surgeon A. G. Lane, the surgeon-in-chief of Winder Hospital, warned one of his surgeons to watch the "Basket Women" from Oregon Hill carefully: "Past experience has established the fact that these women are made the channel of introducing whiskey and improper articles of diet among the sick—You will strictly prohibit these women from entering your Division of the Hospital and when seen anywhere within the limits of the same you will see that your Stewards and Ward Masters place the contents of their baskets (when suitable) upon the Dining Table of your Convalescents" (Lane to surgeon in charge of Winder No. 2, Dec. 17, 1863, Winder Hospital Records, vol. 547: 143).

62. Schroeder-Lein, *Confederate Hospitals on the Move*, 42.

63. Pember, *Southern Woman's Story*, 66.

64. W. A. Davis to McCaw, Feb. 8, 1864, Chimborazo Records, vol. 317: 87.

65. *Richmond Daily Whig*, Sept. 14, 1863.

66. Pember, *Southern Woman's Story*, 43. Discussing the sad plight of Marylanders, Pember observed that, for them, furloughs were impossible—"there was no home that could be reached."

67. S. E. Habersham, order, Chimborazo No. 2, Oct. 15, 1864, Chimborazo Records, vol. 408: 35.

68. Finley P. Curtis, qtd. in Denney, *Civil War Medicine*, 199.

69. Duffy, *From Humors to Medical Science*, 158. These hospitals were established beginning in 1863.

70. Circular, Dec. 4, 1862, Chimborazo Records, vol. 408: 1.

71. Carrington to McCaw, May 24, 1864, Chimborazo Records, vol. 709, 111.
72. Carrington to McCaw, Feb. 10, 1865, Chimborazo Records, vol. 709: 284.
73. Carrington to McCaw, June 7, 1864, Chimborazo Records, vol. 709: 126.
74. N.d., Chimborazo Records, vol. 18: n.p.
75. N.d., Chimborazo Records, vol. 546: 11. The fact that any patients at Chimborazo were allowed into private quarters shows that the patients there were respectable people with at least some monetary resources. This differs significantly from the type of patients found in civilian antebellum hospitals.
76. Moore to Assistant Surgeon W. H. Prileau, medical purveyor, Savannah, Mar. 17, 1863, Surgeon General Office Records, vol. 740: 141.
77. N.d., Chimborazo Records, vol. 18: n.p.
78. Carrington to McCaw, June 23, 1864, Chimborazo Records, vol. 709: 135.
79. Gaillard, circular, Dec. 4, 1862, Chimborazo Records, vol. 408: 1.
80. Carrington to McCaw, Sept. 9, 1863, Chimborazo Records, vol. 708: 217.
81. Carrington to McCaw, Dec. 21, 1864, Chimborazo Records, vol. 709: 251.
82. Moore to McCaw, Mar. 18, 1862, Chimborazo Records, vol. 408: 6. Chimborazo's records show that very few of these types of transfers occurred.
83. W. A. Davis to McCaw, n.d., Chimborazo Records, vol. 317: 3.
84. Death register, Chimborazo Records, vol. 83: n.p.
85. McCaw, order, Apr. 9, 1862, Chimborazo Records: vol. 408: 8.
86. J. Boulware, hospital steward, Sixth South Carolina Volunteers, May 27, 1862, qtd. in Denney, *Civil War Medicine,* 110. Boulware referred to the cemetery as "Oak Grove," but it is clearly Oakwood.
87. Furgurson, *Ashes of Glory,* 155.
88. Pember, *Southern Woman's Story,* 71.
89. Patients to McCaw, Dec. 26, 1862, Chimborazo Records, vol. 707: 246.
90. Carrington to McCaw, June 2, 1864, Chimborazo Records, vol. 709: 119.
91. Carrington to McCaw, Aug. 6, 1863, Chimborazo Records, vol. 708: 189.
92. Philip Whitlock, qtd. in Furgurson, *Ashes of Glory,* 183.
93. W. A. Davis to Brigadier General John Winder, n.d., Chimborazo Records, vol. 317: 56.
94. W. A. Davis to Carrington, Jan. 11, 1864, Chimborazo Records, vol. 317: n.p.
95. W. A. Davis to McCaw, Aug. 5, 1863, Chimborazo Records, vol. 317: 30–31, 36. The records do not reveal why the patient was refusing the operation. An article in the *Confederate States Medical and Surgical Journal* (hereafter *CSMS Journal*) reported another example of a patient who refused to consent to the amputation of his arm; he kept his arm and recovered. See John Stainback Wilson, surgeon, Jackson Hospital, "Resection of Upper-half of Humerus," *CSMS Journal* 1, no. 4 (Apr. 1864): 56; this issue was reprinted as part of a single volume reproducing the entire run of the journal (Metuchen, N.J.: Scarecrow Press, 1976).
96. William A. Davis, surgeon in charge, Chimborazo No. 4, S. E. Habersham, surgeon in charge, Chimborazo No. 2, and E. M. Seabrook, surgeon in charge, Chimborazo No. 5, "Report of cases of Gun-shot Fracture of Femur treated without operative procedure, Chimborazo Hospital," *CSMS Journal* 1, no. 1 (Jan. 1864): 10.
97. M. T. Leadbetter, Company C, Fifth Alabama Battalion, qtd. in Denney, *Civil War Medicine,* 126.
98. Corporal William E. Traher, Company E, Sixth Louisiana Infantry, "Recollections," Sept. 21, 1926, unpublished account; copy in the Chimborazo File, Richmond National Battlefield Park Headquarters.

99. Spencer Glasgow Welch, *A Confederate Surgeon's Letters to His Wife* (Marietta, Ga.: Continental, 1954), 74.

100. Cunningham, *Doctors in Gray,* 53.

101. Cunningham, *Doctors in Gray,* 53.

102. Qtd. in George Worthington Adams, *Doctors in Blue: The Medical History of the Union Army in the Civil War* (New York: Henry Schuman, 1952), 93.

103. Louisa May Alcott, *Hospital Sketches* (1863; rpt. Cambridge, Mass.: Applewood Books, 1986), 89–90.

CHAPTER 5

1. Furgurson, *Ashes of Glory,* 191. Furgurson's comment explained Richmond in 1863; New Orleans was already under Union control.

2. Richard D. Goff, *Confederate Supply* (Durham, N.C.: Duke Univ. Press, 1969), 130.

3. Chimborazo No. 4 to quartermaster, requisition, Aug. 29, 1863, Chimborazo Records, vol. 317: 38.

4. Medical Director Office Records, vol. 469.

5. *The Medical and Surgical History of the Civil War* (1870–88; rpt. Wilmington, N.C.: Broadfoot Publishing Co., 1990), vol. 12: 920. Each field regiment was provided with three hospital tents and one Sibley tent. Hereafter this collection (originally published as *The Medical and Surgical History of the War of the Rebellion*) will be referred to as *Medical and Surgical History.*

6. *Medical and Surgical History,* 12: 920.

7. Carrington to McCaw, June 1, 1864, Chimborazo Records, vol. 709: 118; Carrington to McCaw, May 26, 1864, Chimborazo Records, vol. 709: 112.

8. Major W. G. Bentley, Quartermaster's Department, to McCaw, June 6, 1864, Chimborazo Records, vol. 709: 123.

9. Carrington to McCaw, Sept. 2, 1864, Chimborazo Records, vol. 709: 184.

10. W. A. Davis, Aug. 4, 1863, Chimborazo Records, vol. 317: 37.

11. *Regulations for the Army,* 105.

12. S. E. Habersham, n.d., Chimborazo Records, vol. 408: 25, 26.

13. From a North Carolina infantry bivouac near Fredericksburg to McCaw, Jan. 11, 1862, Chimborazo Records, vol. 707: 29; Moore to McCaw, July 28, 1863, Chimborazo Records, vol. 708: 182.

14. Moore to McCaw, Jan. 7, 1863, Chimborazo Records, vol. 708: 6. Moore's letter was a response to McCaw's request for clothing for Chimborazo's nurses. Moore informed McCaw that the quartermaster did not supply clothing for the nurses.

15. Pember, *Southern Woman's Story,* 60.

16. Winder No. 2 to Carrington, report, Jan. 7, 1864, Winder Records, vol. 547: 153.

17. Furgurson, *Ashes of Glory,* 179.

18. Moore to McCaw, Dec. 5, 1861, Chimborazo Records, vol. 707: 16.

19. Untitled document, Chimborazo File, Richmond National Battlefield Park Headquarters. Obviously a primary source, this single-page document is identified only by the notation "Correspondence, etc. Series 4, vol. III," 1075. This document also stated, "The surgeon in charge of Jackson Hospital has the offer of a contract for wood to be supplied the hospital; the quartermaster refused to make the contract, stating he had made ample provision. At Winder hospital the surgeon in

charge . . . offered, if he was provided with a small number of teams, to supply his own fuel. The quartermaster refused, asserting that he could supply the hospital with the wood required."

20. Davis to McCaw, Jan. 9, 1864, Chimborazo Records, vol. 317, 79; F. Soml, Surgeon General's Office, to McCaw, Jan. 6, 1864, Chimborazo Records, vol. 709, 4; Chimborazo Records, vol. 358: n.p.

21. Pember, *Southern Woman's Story*, 60.

22. Chimborazo Records, vol. 358: n.p. The wood heated 162 fires, 12 of which were for the matrons. The number of patients and attendants at Chimborazo that month was approximately one thousand. The figures for the bushels of coal begin to decline in February 1865, when hospitals in the Richmond area received only 3,575 of the 3,600 bushels requested.

23. John Jackson, acting assistant surgeon, report of the officer of the day, Nov. 3, 1864, Chimborazo Records, vol. 324: n.p.

24. Schroeder-Lein, *Confederate Hospitals on the Move*, 72; James L. Nichols, *The Confederate Quartermaster in the Trans-Mississippi* (Austin, Tex: Univ. of Texas Press, 1964), 6–7.

25. Untitled document, Chimborazo File, 1075.

26. Moore to McCaw, Jan. 30, 1863, Chimborazo Records, vol. 708: n.p.

27. After McCaw wrote to Moore for information about the commutation of quarters and rations for matrons, Moore responded, "[N]o commutation is allowed by law. The matrons [sic] place is at the hospital, and Suitable accommodations should be provided there. The precedent of the allowance of commutations would probably lead to an abuse of the priviledge" (Moore to McCaw, Jan. 30, 1863, Chimborazo Records, vol. 708: n.p.). The monthly funding of rooms for matrons began in September 1864, according to Medical Director Office Records, vol. 469: n.p.

28. Cunningham, *Doctors in Gray*, 146, 155.

29. *Regulations for the Army*, 244–51. Although this regulation was intended to give surgeons more flexibility, it resulted in purveyors having to compete with the army to obtain many of these basic supplies.

30. Medical Purveyor's Office to McCaw, Oct. 15, 1861, Chimborazo Records, vol. 707: 1; Medical Purveyor's Office to McCaw, Mar. 12, 1862, Chimborazo Records, vol. 707: 50.

31. Quartermaster's Department to McCaw, Dec. 7, 1863, Chimborazo Records, vol. 708: 262.

32. Surgeon General's Office to McCaw, Jan. 8, 1864, Chimborazo Records, vol. 709: 5.

33. Surgeons S. E. Habersham and P. F. Browne, board of survey report, Oct. 15, 1864, Chimborazo Records, vol. 709: 207.

34. Surgeons S. E. Habersham and P. F. Browne, board of survey report, Nov. 20, 1864, Chimborazo Records, vol. 709: 228.

35. Duffy, *From Humors to Medical Science*, 165.

36. Cunningham, *Doctors in Gray*, 147–48; Norman H. Franke, "Pharmacy and Pharmacists in the Confederacy," *Georgia Historical Quarterly* 38 (Mar. 1954): 12, 18–22; Byron Stinson, "The Army Disease," *American History Illustrated*, Dec. 1971, 10. Ipecac was used as a strong emetic; foxglove, similar to modern digitalis, helped the patient to develop a stronger heartbeat. For more information, see Alfred Goodman Gilman, Louis S. Goodman, Theodore W. Rall, and Ferid Murad, eds. *The Pharmacological Basis of Therapeutics*, 7th ed. (New York: Macmillan, 1985), 491, 716.

37. Moore to Assistant Surgeon W. H. Prioleau, medical purveyor, Savannah, Mar. 19, 1863, Surgeon General Office Record, vol. 740, 149.
38. Cunningham, *Doctors in Gray,* 148–49. The quotation from Moore appears on page 149.
39. Moore to McCaw, Chimborazo Records, vol. 305: 313.
40. Cunningham, *Doctors in Gray,* 159–60.
41. Cunningham, *Doctors in Gray,* 161.
42. June 1863, Chimborazo Records, vol. 72: 4–5.
43. Moore to Carrington, Feb. 29, 1864, Surgeon General Office Records, vol. 741: 94.
44. Charleston *Mercury,* Nov. 13, 1861, qtd. in Ferguson, *Ashes of Glory,* 101.
45. Moore to Assistant Surgeon W. H. Prioleau, medical purveyor, Savannah, June 11, 1863, Surgeon General Office Records, vol. 740: 359. Another connection between Stearns and Chimborazo was his nearby Tree Hill plantation, where the hospital pastured its cows and goats.
46. Carrington, circular no. 9, July 16, 1864, Chimborazo Records, vol. 7: n.p.
47. Moore, circular no. 10, Nov. 28, 1864, *Confederate Imprints,* 1013.
48. Lafayette Guild, qtd. in Cunningham, *Doctors in Gray,* 158.
49. Cunningham, *Doctors in Gray,* 158.
50. Circular, Sept. 5, 1864, Chimborazo Records, vol. 364: n.p.
51. Apr. 4, 1865, Chimborazo Records, vol. 305: n.p.
52. N.d., Winder Records, vol. 547: 166–67.
53. Carrington to McCaw, May 23, 1863, Chimborazo Records, vol. 708, 141.
54. Carrington to McCaw, Mar. 2, 1865, Chimborazo Records, vol. 709: 294. That same day, Carrington directed McCaw "to throw away none of the Straw now in use until other is obtained" (Carrington to McCaw, Mar. 2, 1865, Chimborazo Records, vol. 709: 295).
55. Moore to Assistant Surgeon W. H. Prioleau, medical purveyor, Savannah, Mar. 28, 1863, Surgeon General Office Records, vol. 740: 179.
56. John H. Claiborne served as the commissary agent at Chimborazo.
57. Cunningham, *Doctors in Gray,* 80–82. Medical regulations in early 1862 stated that the standard ration per soldier per day was as follows: "three-fourths of a pound of pork or bacon, or one and a fourth pounds of fresh or salt beef; eighteen ounces of bread or flour, or twelve ounces of hard bread, or one and a fourth pounds of corn meal; and at the rate, to one hundred rations, of eight quarts of peas or beans, or, in lieu thereof, ten pounds of rice; six pounds of coffee; twelve pounds sugar; four quarts of vinegar; one and a half pounds of tallow, or one and a fourth pounds adamantine, or one pound sperm candles; four pounds of soap, and two quarts of salt" (*Regulations for the Army,* 193). Also, part of the ration of an enlisted man was one pound of tobacco per month, according to a circular dated May 16, 1864 from Moore to the medical directors in the field and hospitals (Chimborazo Records, vol. 9: n.p.). The *Regulations for the Army* (195) further specified that whenever a soldier could not carry his ration with him for some reason, he received the monetary value of the ration (the "commuted" value).
58. S. Cooper, adjutant and inspector general, circular, Dec. 29, 1863, Chimborazo Records, vol. 553: 83.
59. Moore to medical directors of hospitals, circular no. 3, Feb. 27, 1864, Chimborazo Records, vol. 9, n.p.
60. Carrington to McCaw, Feb. 15, 1864, Chimborazo Records, vol. 709: 33.

61. McCaw to all stewards at Chimborazo, Oct. 1, 1863, Chimborazo Records, vol. 708: 230.
62. Nov. 7, 1861, Orange Court House and Farmville Records, vol. 546: 1.
63. George Gates to McCaw, n.d., Chimborazo Records, vol. 709: 346. Gates ran the bakery until December 1864, at which time McCaw began combing Chimborazo's ward for a suitable replacement. See McCaw to S. E. Habersham, circular, Jan. 14, 1865, Chimborazo Records, vol. 18: n.p.
64. McCaw to surgeons in charge, Jan. 21, 1864, Chimborazo Records, vol. 709: 16. On December 4, 1863, flour was selling for $115 a barrel on the streets of Richmond, although it was slightly cheaper at the commissary, according to diarist Mary Chesnut (*Mary Chesnut's Civil War*, 498).
65. Pember, *Southern Woman's Story*, 58–59.
66. Chimborazo Records, vol. 307: n.p.
67. Records of Chimborazo's bakeries, Chimborazo Records, vol. 638; Pember, *Southern Woman's Story*, 137.
68. H. B. Gaines to McCaw, Oct. 20, 1863, Chimborazo Records, vol. 708: 246. In this letter, Gaines asked McCaw whether he should purchase soap. Chimborazo No. 5 had none on hand and could get none from Miles, even though, according to the bakery's books, Miles owed them some thirteen hundred pounds of soap. Gaines had offered him forty pounds of grease to make some more, but Miles refused to take it until he had access to sixty more pounds, arguing that it cost the same to make a hundred pounds as ten pounds. This letter is a good example of the smaller issues at Chimborazo that McCaw and his surgeons had to address.
69. Moore to Samuel Stout, Sept. 26, 1864, *Confederate Imprints*, 1050.
70. Furgurson, *Ashes of Glory*, 182.
71. Charles W. Arnold to McCaw, Jan. 20, 1863, Chimborazo Records, vol. 708: n.p.
72. Carrington to McCaw, Aug. 11, 1863, Chimborazo Records, vol. 708: 192. Apparently, the competition between hospitals' purchasing agents was not limited to the Richmond area. In *Confederate Hospitals on the Move* (114), Glenna Schroeder-Lein noted that it occurred in Samuel Stout's hospitals as well.
73. Moore, circular no. 15, Aug. 10, 1864, *Confederate Imprints*, 998.
74. Thomas Scott to McCaw, Dec. 16, 1862, Chimborazo Records, vol. 305: n.p.
75. "Of Chimborazo Park." Chimborazo's records provide a list of the property belonging to Chimborazo Hospital that had been destroyed by Sheridan's Raiding on March 10, 1865. A boat and tram top the full-page list, which included various items such as cotton cloth and food. The cost of the damage was estimated at $15,339. See Chimborazo Records, vol. 80: 315.
76. Cunningham, *Doctors in Gray*, 52.
77. Carrington to McCaw, Oct. 4, 1864, Chimborazo Records, vol. 709: 201.
78. Furgurson, *Ashes of Glory*, 294, 310.
79. Schroeder-Lein, *Confederate Hospitals on the Move*, 114.
80. Tobias G. Richardson, assistant medical director (field) of the Army of Tennessee, to Samuel H. Stout, medical director of hospitals for the Army of Tennessee, Mar. 1864, qtd. in Schroeder-Lein, *Confederate Hospitals on the Move*, 120.
81. McCaw to Sergeant Yarrington, Oct. 1, 1863, Chimborazo Records, vol. 708: 231.
82. Notice from McCaw, Oct. 3, 1863, Chimborazo Records, vol. 708: 234.
83. Moore, circular, Dec. 2, 1863, Chimborazo Records, vol. 553: 83.
84. Carrington, circular, Oct. 1, 1863, Chimborazo Records, vol. 7: n.p.

85. H. B. Gaines to McCaw, Oct. 20, 1863, Chimborazo Records, vol. 708: 246.
86. Moore to McCaw, Feb. 18, 1863, Chimborazo Records, vol. 708: 53.
87. Moore to McCaw, Feb. 5, 1863, Chimborazo Records, vol. 708: n.p.
88. Surgeon General's Office, circular, Dec. 23, 1863, Chimborazo Records, vol. 553: 82.
89. Carrington to McCaw, July 29, 1864, Chimborazo Records, vol. 709: 160.
90. Moore to McCaw, Mar. 3, 1863, Chimborazo Records, vol. 708, 58. The sales of offal from Chimborazo also went into the post fund. When Moore approved McCaw's proposal, he added, "As this is a separate post, the profits of the bakery can be used according to regulations."
91. Untitled document, Chimborazo File, 1075.
92. McCaw, qtd. in "Of Chimborazo Park." The article further noted, "Mr. Meminger, Secretary of the C.S. Treasury agreed to pay in gold on the 29th of March, and on the 3rd day of April the city of Richmond surrendered."
93. McCaw, qtd. in "Of Chimborazo Park."
94. Carrington to McCaw, May 27, 1864, Chimborazo Records, vol. 709: 114.
95. O. F. Manson, medical agent of the state of North Carolina, to McCaw, June 17, 1864, Chimborazo Records, vol. 709: 132.
96. William Quentin Maxwell, *Lincoln's Fifth Wheel: The Political History of the United States Sanitary Commission* (New York: Longmans, Green, & Co., 1956), 9. The USSC, the U.S. Christian Commission, and the Western Sanitary Commission together raised over fifty million dollars in contributions, according to Nina Bennett Smith ("The Women Who Went To The War: The Union Army Nurse in the Civil War" [Ph. D. diss., Northwestern Univ., 1981], 2).
97. *Richmond Daily Whig,* Sept. 14. 1863; see also Chimborazo Records, vol. 709: 344.
98. Pember, *Southern Woman's Story,* 40.
99. General Hospital No. 24 Records, Record Group 109, War Department Collection of Confederate Records, National Archives, Washington, D.C., vol. 172.
100. Chesnut, *Mary Chesnut's Civil War,* 155.
101. Chesnut, *Mary Chesnut's Civil War,* 195.
102. Chesnut, *Mary Chesnut's Civil War,* 217.
103. Chesnut, *Mary Chesnut's Civil War,* 133 (quotation), 158.
104. "Remarks" in morning report, July 17, 1862, Chimborazo Records, vol. 321: 118, 132, 208.
105. Pember, *Southern Woman's Story,* 98.

CHAPTER 6

1. McPherson, *Ordeal by Fire,* 383.
2. Peter J. Parish, *The American Civil War* (New York: Holmes & Meier, 1975), 147, qtd. in McPherson, *Ordeal by Fire,* 383.
3. McPherson, *Ordeal by Fire,* 384.
4. Carrington to McCaw, Feb. 29, 1864, Chimborazo Records, vol. 709: 44.
5. Carrington to McCaw, Feb. 20, 1865, Chimborazo Records, vol. 709: 288; Carrington, circular, Mar. 11, 1865, Chimborazo Records, vol. 7: 9.
6. Carrington to McCaw, Jan. 17, 1865, Chimborazo Records, vol. 709: 216.
7. Blanton, *Medicine in Virginia,* 54.
8. Samuel Preston Moore, qtd. in Russell V. Bowers, "A Confederate General Hospital: Chimborazo Post (1862–1865)," *The Scarab,* Nov. 1962, 3.

9. Carrington to "Sir," Mar. 14, 1864, *Confederate Imprints,* microfilm, 1065-1.

10. Staff Record Book, Feb. 29, 1864, Chimborazo Records, vol. 317: 93; Carrington to McCaw, Feb. 19, 1864, Chimborazo Records, vol. 709: 33.

11. Oct. 22, 1862, Chimborazo Records, vol. 707: 191; Moore to McCaw, Nov. 1, 1862, Chimborazo Records, vol. 707: 209.

12. Moore to McCaw, June 17, 1863, Chimborazo Records, vol. 708: 159.

13. Moore to McCaw, Jan. 8, 1864, Chimborazo Records, vol. 709: 6.

14. Pember, *A Southern Woman's Story,* 49.

15. Carrington to McCaw, Mar. 7, 1864, Chimborazo Records, vol. 709: 53.

16. William D. Sharpe, introduction to *CSMS Journal* (1864–65; rpt. Metuchen, N.J.: Scarecrow Press, 1976), v.

17. "Salutatory," *CSMS Journal* 1, no. 1 (Jan. 1864): 13.

18. Carrington to McCaw, Nov. 8, 1864, Chimborazo Records, vol. 709: 223.

19. Nov. 21, 1863, Chimborazo Records, vol. 708: 259.

20. "The Prospect before Us," *CSMS Journal* 1, no. 5 (May 1864): 78.

21. "Editorial and Miscellaneous," *CSMS Journal* 2, no. 1 (Jan. 1865): 11.

22. Sharpe, introduction to *CSMS Journal,* v.

23. *The Lancet* (Apr. 16, 1864), cited in Sharpe, introduction to *CSMS Journal,* ix.

24. Sharpe, introduction to *CSMS Journal,* ix–xi.

25. William A. Davis to E. M. Seabrook, Feb. 9, 1864, Chimborazo Records, vol. 709: 28.

26. "Association of Army and Navy Surgeons," *CSMS Journal* 1, no. 1 (Jan. 1864): 14.

27. "Association of Army and Navy Surgeons," 15–16.

28. "Association of Army and Navy Surgeons," 15.

29. "Association of Army and Navy Surgeons," 16.

30. *Medical and Surgical History,* 5: 29. Nine hundred ninety-eight patients deserted. The fate of the other 26,501 patients is unknown: 14,464 were transferred to other hospitals, 5,537 were furloughed, and no record of disposition was found for the remaining 6,500.

31. S. E. Habersham, order, June 11, 1864, Chimborazo Records, vol. 408: 33.

32. Carrington to McCaw, June 1, 1864, Chimborazo Records, vol. 709: 118; Carrington to McCaw, June 3, 1864, Chimborazo Records, vol. 709: 121; McCaw to Carrington, June 22, 1864, Chimborazo Records, vol. 709: 134.

33. W. A. Davis, order, Mar. 25, 1864, Chimborazo Records, vol. 317: 101.

34. Carrington to McCaw, Mar. 13, 1865, Chimborazo Records, vol. 709: 303.

35. Julian E. Kuz and Bradley P. Bengtson, *Orthopaedic Injuries of the Civil War: An Atlas on Orthopaedic Injuries and Treatments During the Civil War* (Kennesaw, Ga.: Kennesaw Mountain Press, 1996), 42.

36. Blustein, *Preserve Your Love for Science,* 71.

37. Surgeon General's Office, circular, July 6, 1863, Winder Hospital Records, vol. 547: 77.

38. Carrington, circular, June 2, 1864, Chimborazo Records, vol. 7: 7.

39. Carrington to McCaw, Jan. 28, 1864, Chimborazo Records, vol. 709: 18.

40. Thomas D. Brock, Michael T. Madigan, John M. Martinko, and Jack Parker, *Biology of Microorganisms,* 7th ed. (Englewood Cliffs, N.J.: Prentice Hall, 1994), 19.

41. John Harley Warner, "The Fall and Rise of Professional Mystery," *The Laboratory Revolution in Medicine,* ed. Andrew Cunningham and Perry Williams (New York: Cambridge Univ. Press, 1992), 121.

42. Charles E. Rosenberg, *The Care of Strangers: The Rise of America's Hospital System* (New York: Basic, 1987), 82.

43. Andrew Cunningham, "Transforming Plague," in *Laboratory Revolution in Medicine*, ed. Cunningham and Williams, 217–19.
44. Cunningham, "Transforming Plague," 22–-22.
45. Cunningham, "Transforming Plague," 223.
46. *Medical and Surgical History*, 5: 111.
47. John Hughes Bennet, M.D., "The Natural Progress of Disease," *CSMS Journal* 1:6 (June 1864): 96.
48. Bennet, "Natural Progress of Disease," 96.
49. Cunningham, *Doctors in Gray*, 163–83.
50. *Medical and Surgical History*, 3: 1.
51. Joseph Jones, Surgeon, qtd. in Cunningham, *Doctors in Gray*, 185–86.
52. Cunningham, *Doctors in Gray*, 185.
53. *Medical and Surgical History*, 3: 2.
54. The authors of the *Medical and Surgical History* strongly supported this statement in their analysis and discussion of the statistics.
55. *Medical and Surgical History*, 4: 483.
56. Cunningham, *Doctors in Gray*, 187.
57. Cunningham, *Doctors in Gray*, 185.
58. Cunningham, *Doctors in Gray*, 207.
59. Cunningham, *Doctors in Gray*, 208.
60. *Medical and Surgical History*, 5: 111.
61. Samuel Logan, "Prophylactic Effects of Quinine," *CSMS Journal* 1, no. 6 (June 1864): 1; Cunningham, *Doctors in Gray*, 193.
62. Patient Register of Howard's Grove Hospital, Howard's Grove Records, vol. 192.
63. S. E. Habersham to McCaw, July 22, 1864, reply to Carrington to McCaw, July 21, 1864, Chimborazo Records, vol. 709: 153.
64. Surgeon General's Office, circular, Dec. 1862, Orange Court House and Farmville Records, vol. 546: 83.
65. W. A. Davis to McCaw, Feb. 9, 1864, Chimborazo Records, vol. 317: 88.
66. Surgeon General's Office, circular, Oct. 16, 1863, Chimborazo Records, vol. 7: 9.
67. Habersham, order, June 23, 1864, Chimborazo Records, vol. 408: 35.
68. Surgeon General's Office, circular, Apr. 12, 1864, Chimborazo Records, vol. 7: 7.
69. Cunningham, *Doctors in Gray*, 198.
70. O. Kratz, surgeon, "On Vaccination and Variolous Diseases," *CSMS Journal* 1, no. 7 (July 1864): 104.
71. Cunningham, *Doctors in Gray*, 197.
72. Surgeon General's Office, Circular No. 2, Feb. 6, 1864.
73. J. C. M. Merillat, surgeon, "On the Absense of Chlorides in the Urine of Persons affected with Variolous Diseases," *CSMS Journal* 1, no 5 (May 1864): 70.
74. Merillat, "On the Absence of Chlorides in the Urine," 71.
75. *Medical and Surgical History* 6: 719. Catarrh is defined as "the excessive secretion of thick phlegm or mucus by the mucous membrane of the nose, nasal sinuses, nasopharynx, or air passages" (*Bantam Medical Dictionary* [New York: Bantam Books, 1981], 67).
76. *Medical and Surgical History*, 6: 757.
77. *Medical and Surgical History*, 6: 751–52.
78. *Medical and Surgical History*, 6: 808. Asthenia refers to weakness or loss of strength, according to the *Bantam Medical Dictionary* (32).

79. *Medical and Surgical History,* 6: 806–7, 809.

80. *Medical and Surgical History,* 6: 819–20, 828.

81. Alfred J. Bollet, "How Good or Bad Was Medical Care during the Civil War?" (presentation at the National Museum of Civil War Medicine, Fredericksburg, Md., Aug. 1995); Dr. P. W. Douglas, "Tartarized Antimony in Traumatic Pneumonia and Pleuritis" (record of percussion and auscultation), *CSMS Journal* 1, no. 9 (Sept. 1864): 136.

82. Jno. H. Claiborne, surgeon in charge of Petersburg Hospitals, "On the use of Phytolacca Decandra in Camp Itch," *CSMS Journal* 1, no. 3 (Mar. 1864): 39.

83. S. R. Chambers, assistant surgeon, "On the Treatment of Camp Itch," *CSMS Journal* 1, no. 1 (Jan. 1865): 10. Chambers asserted that in over one hundred cases this treatment had never failed him.

84. Moore to McCaw, Jan. 29, 1862, Chimborazo Records, vol. 707: 33.

85. Carrington to McCaw, Aug. 24, 1864, Chimborazo Records, vol. 709: 175.

86. *CSMS Journal,* 1, no. 1 (Jan. 1864): 8.

87. Pember, *Southern Woman's Story,* 63.

88. S. E. Habersham, order, Apr. 2, 1865, Chimborazo Records, vol. 408: 36.

89. Pember, *Southern Woman's Story,* 39.

90. J. J. Chisolm, *A Manual of Military Surgery,* Confederate States of America Surgeon General's Office, 1863, cited in James O. Breeden, "Confederate General Hospitals: The Front Line of the South's Civil War Health Care System," *North Carolina Medical Journal* 53, no. 2 (Feb. 1992): 115.

91. Chisolm, cited in Breeden, "Hospitals," 116.

92. "Eleven Cases of Compound Fracture of Cranium by Gunshot Wound treated at Chimborazo Hospital," *CSMS Journal* 1, no. 4 (Apr. 1864): 57.

93. "Eleven Cases of Compound Fracture," 57.

94. P. F. Browne, "Gun-Shot Wound of the Chest Treated by Hermetically Sealing," *CSMS Journal* 1, no. 10 (Oct. 1864): 163.

95. T. Longmore, deputy inspector general and professor of military surgery, Army Medical School, "Remarks on the Recently Proposed American Plan of Treating Gun-Shot Wounds of the Chest by 'Hermetically Sealing,'" *London Lancet,* Mar. 1864, reprinted in *CSMS Journal* 1, no. 4 (Apr. 1864): 63; J. J. Chisolm, Confederate surgeon, "Conversion of Gun-Shot Wounds into Incised Wounds as a means of Speedy Cure," *CSMS Journal* 1, no. 9 (Sept. 1864): 138; James Brown McCaw, surgeon in chief, Chimborazo Hospital, "On the Treatment of Gun-Shot Wounds by 'Hermetically Sealing,'" *CSMS Journal* 1, no. 9 (Sept. 1864): 138; B. Howard, cited in Longmore, "Remarks," 63.

96. Captain Claude E. Minié of the French army designed this bullet in the 1840s. Its elongated cartridge contained an iron or wooden plug in its base that expanded when fired, allowing it to be easily loaded and used in a rifled barrel. Because Minié's design was expensive to produce, an American, James H. Burton, changed the base of the projectile from a plug to a cavity that expanded from the gas created by the powder explosion and thus developed the "minié ball" used frequently in Springfield and Enfield rifles on both sides during the American Civil War. The minié ball greatly expanded the range of the rifle. The effective range of a smoothbore musket was approximately 80 yards, while that of a rifle with a minié ball reached about 400 yards. The maximum ranges of muskets and rifles were 250 and 1,000 yards, respectively. See McPherson, *Ordeal by Fire,* 194; Sharpe, introduction to *CSMS Journal,* viii.

97. Duffy, *From Humors to Medical Science,* 161; Breeden, "Confederate General Hospitals," 115.
98. Simon Baruch, *Reminiscences of a Confederate Surgeon,* qtd. in Breeden, "Confederate General Hospitals," 115.
99. *Military and Surgical History,* 12: 868.
100. *Military and Surgical History,* 12: 761.
101. *Military and Surgical History,* 12: 866–67.
102. Moore to Medical Director to McCaw, Oct. 1, 1862, Chimborazo Records, vol. 707: 179.
103. G. M. B. Maughs, "Thoughts on Surgery, Operative and Conservative, suggested by a visit to the Battle-field and Hospitals of the Army of Tennessee," *CSMS Journal* 1, no. 9 (Sept. 1864): 130–31.
104. Prof. Skey, surgeon, St. Bartholomew's Hospital, abridged by Frank A. Ramsay, medical director, "Local Injuries Justifying the Amputation of a Limb," *CSMS Journal* 2, no. 1 (Jan. 1865): 5.
105. Medical Case Record, n.d., Chimborazo Records, vol. 97: n.p. The patient served in Duke Co. K, Seventeenth Mississippi Regiment. He was admitted on May 6, 1863. The case record ends on a positive note, but no further record indicates whether the patient survived.
106. F. William Blaisdell, "Medical Advances during the Civil War," *Archives of Surgery* 123 (1988): 1049.
107. Cold-water dressings were seen as "invaluable in the treatment of gunshot wounds" (J. B. Read, "Cold Water Dressings," *CSMS Journal* 1, no. 6 [June 1864]: 92).
108. Read, "Cold Water Dressings," 92.
109. Read, "Cold Water Dressings," 92.
110. Russell Murdock, "On the Application of Smith's Anterior Splint," *CSMS Journal* 1:5 (May 1864): 71–72. Professor N. R. Smith of Baltimore invented this popular apparatus.
111. Prescription Book, Aug. 1863–July 1864, Chimborazo Records, vol. 496: n.p. Williams's treatment was first recorded on June 22, 1864; he died on July 24.
112. "Statistics of Chimborazo Hospital from Nov. 1, 1861, to Nov. 1, 1863," *CSMS Journal* 1, no. 1 (Jan. 1864): 8. The reader should remember that these figures were computed without considering the number of patients transferred.
113. Kuz and Bengtson, *Orthopaedic Injuries of the Civil War,* 15.
114. Thomas Watson, *Lectures on the Principles and Practice of Physic* (Philadelphia: Blanchard & Lea, 1858), 113. Watson's work was a printed series of lectures he delivered at King's College in London.
115. Watson, *Lectures,* 115.
116. J. S. Billings, Surgeon General's Office, Circular no. 2: A Report on Excisions of the Head of the Femur for Gunshot Injury (Washington, D.C.: Government Printing Office, 1869), in Kuz and Bengtson, *Orthopaedic Injuries,* 16.
117. Robert Berkow, ed., *The Merck Manual of Diagnosis and Therapy,* 15th ed. (Rahway, N. J.: Merck Sharp & Dohme Research Laboratories, 1987), 5. Hereafter this source will be referred to as *Merck Manual.*
118. *Medical and Surgical History,* 12: 824. According to this same source, 2.2 percent of the total gangrene cases among the Union wounded involved head, face, or neck wounds, while 8.2 percent involved wounds to the trunk. Of those with wounds to

the extremities, 844 gangrene cases affected the upper extremities, while 1,522 cases developed gangrene in their lower-extremity wounds. In the Union army, 2,642 cases of gangrene were reported, of which 1,361 cases recovered, and 1,142 died—a mortality rate of 45.6 percent. The remaining 139 cases remained undetermined.

119. *Medical and Surgical History,* 12: 823. This work cited an 1871 article on gangrene by Joseph Jones ("Investigations upon the Nature, Causes, and Treatment of Hospital Gangrene as it prevailed in the Confederate Armies, 1861–1865," in *United States Sanitary Commission Memoirs,* 2nd Surgical Volume [New York, 1871], 174). Jones's article could not be obtained for review. It should be noted that modern physicians do not specifically know the etiology of hospital gangrene, whose contagious nature in the nineteenth century seemed to exceed that of gangrene cases that develop today.

120. Blaisdell, "Medical Advances," 1049.

121. W. W. Keen, acting assistant surgeon for the Union army.

122. Kate Cumming, qtd. in Cunningham, *Doctors in Gray,* 239.

123. Cunningham, *Doctors in Gray,* 239.

124. Keen, qtd. in *Medical and Surgical History* 12: 828.

125. *Merck Manual,* 98–103. quote 102.

126. Keen, qtd. in *Medical and Surgical History,* vol. 12: 829. Keen, a prominent surgeon assigned to a Philadelphia hospital, also used fresh bandages for all the cases, dressed infected wounds last, and encouraged hand-washing between cases. See Blaisdell, "Medical Advances," 1050.

127. Hargrove Hinkley, Confederate surgeon, "Treatment of Hospital Gangrene," *CSMS Journal* 1, no. 1 (Jan. 1864): 131; case of Sam Williams, prescription book, General Hospital No. 24, Richmond, Chimborazo Records, vol. 496.

128. Keen, qtd. in *Medical and Surgical History,* vol. 12: 828.

129. A. G. Lane to surgeon in charge, Winder No. 2, n.d., Winder Records, vol. 547: 245.

130. T. M. Earnhart, qtd. in Denney, *Civil War Medicine,* 303.

131. Earnhart, qtd. in Denney, *Civil War Medicine,* 303.

132. *Medical and Surgical History* 12: 851. Today, erysipelas, a bacterial infection of the skin, is described as a "superficial cellulitis caused by [streptococcus pyogenes]. . . . The lesion is well demarcated, shiny, red, edematous, and tender . . . high fever, chills, and malaise are common" (*Merck Manual,* 2265).

133. *Medical and Surgical History,* 12: 853–55.

134. *Medical and Surgical History,* 12: 855.

135. Prescription book, Apr. 1864, Chimborazo Records, vol. 619: 10.

136. *Medical and Surgical History,* 12: 855.

137. *Merck Manual,* 50.

138. *Merck Manual,* 21–22.

139. *Medical and Surgical History,* vol. 12: 857–58.

140. *Medical and Surgical History,* vol. 12: 858.

141. *Merck Manual,* 64–65.

142. Pember, *Southern Woman's Story,* 76.

143. *Medical and Surgical History,* 12: 818.

144. *Medical and Surgical History,* 12: 820.

145. Blaisdell, "Medical Advances," 1049.

146. *Medical and Surgical History,* 12: 819–23.

147. *Merck Manual,* 99.

148. *Merck Manual,* 100–101.
149. *Medical and Surgical History,* 12: 867.
150. Pember, *Southern Woman's Story,* 61.

CHAPTER 7

1. Both qtd. in Cunningham, *Doctors in Gray,* 269.
2. Jefferson Davis, qtd. in Isobel Stevenson, "American Medicine During the Sixties," *Ciba Symposia* 3 (July 1941): 902.
3. Pember, *Southern Woman's Story,* 91.
4. John Jackson, acting assistant surgeon, report of the officer of the day, Jan. 13, 1865, Chimborazo Records, vol. 324: n.p.
5. E. S. Harrison, report of the officer of the day, Mar. 7, Mar. 19, and Mar. 21, 1865, Chimborazo Records, vol. 324: n.p.
6. Carrington to McCaw, Mar. 14, 1865, Chimborazo Records, vol. 709: 304.
7. Captain F. F. Myer to Major B. P. Nolan, Chief Commissary, state of Virginia, Mar. 13, 1865, copy sent to McCaw, Chimborazo Records, vol. 709: 305.
8. Carrington to McCaw, Mar. 21, 1865, Chimborazo Records, vol. 709: 310.
9. Furgurson, *Ashes of Glory,* 311.
10. Furgurson, *Ashes of Glory,* 304.
11. Furgurson, *Ashes of Glory,* 306.
12. Furgurson, *Ashes of Glory,* 313.
13. H. E. Wood, qtd. in Furgurson, *Ashes of Glory,* 317.
14. Furgurson, *Ashes of Glory,* 320–38. Major General Godfrey Weitzel formally accepted the city's surrender at City Hall at 8:15 that morning.
15. Pember, *Southern Woman's Story,* 98.
16. Furgurson, *Ashes of Glory,* 340.
17. McCaw, qtd. in "Of Chimborazo Park."
18. Pember, *Southern Woman's Story,* 98.
19. Pember, *Southern Woman's Story,* 98.
20. Pember, *Southern Woman's Story,* 100.
21. Pember, *Southern Woman's Story,* 101.
22. Pember, *Southern Woman's Story,* 103.
23. Pember, *Southern Woman's Story,* 103. The supplies at Camp Jackson were supplemented by the United States Sanitary Commission and the Christian Commission. These charitable groups daily received and filled orders signed by the division surgeons and approved by the surgeon-in-charge. J. M. Rand served as the Confederate surgeon-in-charge at Camp Jackson; L. Quick, U.S.V., was his Union counterpart at the facility. See J. M. Rand to surgeons in charge of divisions, Apr. 6, 1865, Winder Records, vol. 547: 276; L. Quick, surgeon in charge, U.S. Volunteers, order, Apr. 14, 1865, *Winder Records,* vol. 547, 282.
24. M. Jennie Armstrong to Rev. William George Hawkins, June 3, 1865, in the *National Freedman* 1:5 (June 1865): 154–55. "Report of Chimborazo Schools, Richmond, Va., From October 9, 1865, to Nov. 1, 1865," *National Freedman* 1, no. 11 (Dec. 1865); "Report of Edward Barker on his visit to City Point and Richmond," *National Freedman* 1, no. 10 (Nov. 1865).

25. J. F. Williams to Rev. Mr. Hawkins, Dec. 30, 1865, published as "The Chimborazo School," *The National Freedman* 2, no. 1 (Jan. 15, 1866): 15.
26. Williams, "The Chimborazo School," 15.
27. R. M. Maney to Rev. W. G. Hawkins, Feb. 2, 1866, published as "Chimborazo," *The National Freedman* 2, no. 2 (Feb. 15, 1866): 61.
28. Maney, "Chimborazo," 61.
29. Miss I. G. Campbell, letter, Feb. 1, 1866, published in *The National Freedman* 2, no. 2 (Feb. 15, 1866): 61.
30. L. E. Williams, "Chimborazo," *The National Freedman* 2, no. 5 (May 15, 1866): 146. One of the supporting agencies of the school was the American Missionary Association.
31. Maney, "Chimborazo," 60.
32. "Beer, Not Wine."
33. "Of Chimborazo Park."
34. "Beer, Not Wine." Erwin E. Ellington, a Richmond citizen and the grandson of Joseph Bacher, was quoted in this article as saying, " A heavy bomb would undoubtedly crash through the few feet of earth above them, and destroy both the vaults and their inhabitants."
35. Judith L. Anthis, "Chimborazo Hospital," Jan. 9, 1985, unpublished compilation of information from Chimborazo file, Richmond National Battlefield Park Headquarters.
36. Rutkow, "Samuel Preston Moore," xiii.
37. Rutkow, "Samuel Preston Moore," xii–xiv.
38. Pember, *Southern Woman's Story*, 103.
39. Bell Irvin Wiley, introduction to *Southern Woman's Story*, by Pember, 12.
40. Blanton, *Medicine in Virginia*, 61. According to his 1994 presentation, "Chimborazo Hospital," Dr. Charles Cook believes this incident to be the beginning of the gentlemen's agreement in place between Richmond's police department and the emergency room of the Medical College of Virginia's University Hospital that survives even today. Dr. Cook is a Richmond physician and retired member of the MCV faculty.
41. Blanton, *Medicine in Virginia*, 81, 100, 120–21, 209, 215, 216, 258.
42. Cook, "Chimborazo Hospital."
43. "James Brown McCaw, M.D.," *The British Medical Journal* 2 (Sept. 8, 1906): 601. This obituary also stated that "For many years he was President of the Mozart Society of Richmond, and it is said that few did more to stimulate interest in music and art in his native city than he." Dr. Charles Cook ("Chimborazo Hospital") noted that only two other physicians associated with the Medical College of Virginia have received the honor of an obituary in this journal: Hunter Holmes McGuire and David Hume.
44. Reprinted in 1990 as the *Medical and Surgical History of the Civil War*.

CHAPTER 8

1. Bollet, *Civil War Medicine*, 217.

Bibliography

Primary Sources

Archives

Collection of the Boston Athanaeum, Boston, Mass.
Confederate Imprints. Microfilmed copies of official publications of the Confederate government. 1955.
National Archives and Records Administration, Washington, D.C.
Record Group 109, War Department Collection of Confederate Records, Chapter 6, Medical Records
    Chimborazo Records, 138 Volumes
    Records from Various Hospitals (Howard's Grove, Jackson, Orange Court House, Farmville, General Hospital No. 24), 12 Volumes
    Medical Department Records, 36 Volumes
    Medical Director's Office Records, 17 Volumes
    Surgeon General's Office Records, 3 Volumes
    Winder Records, 6 Volumes
Richmond National Battlefield Park Headquarters, Richmond, Va.
Chimborazo File
    Anthis, Judith L. "Chimborazo Hospital." Jan. 9, 1985. Unpublished compilation of information.
    "Beer, Not Wine, First Stored in Chimborazo Park Cellars." July 3, 1941. Clipping from unidentified Richmond newspaper.
    Brewer, S. J. G., Company I, Eighth Georgia Infantry. Letters to his wife: Nov. 13, 1861, Dec. 5, 1861, Oct. 20, 1862, Sept. 3, 1862.
    "Of Chimborazo Park." Aug. 8, 1897. Clipping from unidentified Richmond newspaper.
    Traher, Corporal William E., Company E, Sixth Louisiana Infantry. "Recollections." Sept. 21, 1926. Unpublished account.

Books and Articles

Alcott, Louisa May. *Hospital Sketches*. 1863. Reprint, Cambridge, Mass.: Applewood Books, 1986.

Bayard, Robert. *Evidences of the Delusions of Homeopathy*. Saint John, New Brunswick: William Avery, 1857.

Beecher, Catherine E. *A Treatise on Domestic Economy, for the Use of Young Ladies at Home and at School*. New York: Harper & Brothers, 1852.

Bowditch, Henry I. *Public Hygiene in America*. 1877. Reprint, New York: Arno Press, 1972.

"Careless Disinfection." *The Popular Science Monthly* 2 (Nov. 1872): 122.

Chisolm, J. Julian. *A Manual of Military Surgery.* Richmond, Va.: West & Johnston, 1862.

Confederate States Medical and Surgical Journal. Jan. 1864–Mar. 1865. Reprinted in one volume, with an introduction by William D. Sharpe. Metuchen, N.J.: Scarecrow Press, 1976.

Davis, Nicholas A. *The Campaign from Texas to Maryland with the Battle of Fredericksburg.* 1863. Reprint, Austin, Tex.: Steck Co., 1961.

"Furniture for the Sick Room." *Scribner's Monthly* 5 (Feb. 1873): 510–11.

Hospital Plans: Five Essays Relating to the Construction, Organization & Management of Hospitals, Contributed by their Authors for the use of the Johns Hopkins Hospital of Baltimore. New York: William Wood & Co., 1875.

Lane, Alexander. "Address to the Association of Army and Navy Surgeons of the Confederacy." *Southern Practitioner* 26 (1904): 34–41.

Livermore, Mary A. *My Story of the War: A Woman's Narrative of Four Years of Personal Experience.* Hartford, Conn.: A. D. Worthington Co., 1889.

The Medical and Surgical History of the Civil War. 12 vols. 1870–88. Reprint, Wilmington, N.C.: Broadfoot Publishing Co., 1990. Originally published as *The Medical And Surgical History of the War of the Rebellion.*

"The Pleasures of Illness." *Harper's New Monthly Magazine* 1 (1850): 698.

Regulations for the Army of the Confederate States, By Order of the Surgeon General. 1862. Reprint, with a preface, "Samuel Preston Moore," by Ira M. Rutkow, San Francisco: Norman Publishing, 1992.

"The Sick Room." *Scribner's Monthly* 5 (Nov. 1872): 127-28.

Stille, Charles J. *The History of the United States Sanitary Commission: The General Report of Its Work During the War of the Rebellion.* Philadelphia: J. B. Lippincott, 1866.

The War of the Rebellion: A Compilation of the Official Records of the Union and Confederate Armies. 128 vols. Washington, D.C.: Government Printing Office, 1880–1901.

Watson, Thomas. *Lectures on the Principles and Practice of Physic.* Philadelphia: Blandhard & Lea, 1858.

Wilson, Johnathan Stainback. "Health Department." *Godey's Lady's Book* 63 (1861): 534–35.

NEWSPAPERS

"Chimborazo Hospital." *Richmond Whig*, Nov. 1, 1861.

National Freedman. Excerpts from vol. 1, no. 5 (June 1865); vol. 1, no. 10 (Nov. 1865); vol. 1, no. 11 (Dec. 1865); vol. 2, no. 1 (Jan. 15, 1866); vol. 2, no. 2 (Feb. 15, 1866); vol. 2, no. 5 (May 15, 1866).

Richmond Daily Whig, Sept. 14, 1863, and July 7, 1864.

SECONDARY SOURCES

BOOKS AND ARTICLES

Adams, George Worthington. "Confederate Medicine." *Journal of Southern History* 6 (Jan. 1940): 151–66.

———. *Doctors in Blue: The Medical History of the Union Army in the Civil War.* New York: Henry Schuman, 1952.

Bantam Medical Dictionary. New York: Bantam Books, 1981.

Beller, Susan Provost. *Medical Practices in the Civil War.* Cincinnati: Betterway Books, 1992.

Berkow, Robert, ed.. *The Merck Manual of Diagnosis and Therapy.* 15th ed. Rahway, N.J.: Merck Sharp & Dohme Research Laboratories, 1987.

Blackford, Susan Lee. "Susan Blackford Nurses the Wounded at Lynchburg." *The Blue and the Gray: The Story of the Civil War as told by Participants.* Edited by Henry Steele Commager. 1950. Reprint, New York: Fairfax, 1991, 780–82.

Blaisdell, F. William. "Medical Advances during the Civil War." *Archives of Surgery* 123 (1988): 1040–50.

Blanton, Wyndham B. *Medicine in Virginia in the Nineteenth Century.* Richmond, Va.: Garrett & Massie, 1933.

Bloomberg, Susan E., Mary Frank Fox, Robert M. Warner, and Sam Bass Warner Jr. " A Census Probe into Nineteenth-Century Family History: Southern Michigan, 1850–1880." *Journal of Social History* 5 (Fall 1971): 26–45.

Blustein, Bonnie Ellen. *Preserve Your Love For Science: Life of William A. Hammond, American Neurologist.* Cambridge: Cambridge Univ. Press, 1991.

Boardman, Andrew. "An Essay on the Means of Improving Medical Education and Elevating Medical Character." In *Medical America in the Nineteenth Century: Readings from the Literature,* edited by Gert H. Brieger. Baltimore: Johns Hopkins Univ. Press, 1972.

Bollett, Alfred Jay. *Civil War Medicine: Challenges and Triumphs.* Tucson, Ariz.: Galen, 2002.

———. "Scurvy, Sprue, and Starvation: Major Nutritional Deficiency Syndromes During the Civil War." Parts 1 and 2. *Medical Times* 117 (Nov. 1989): 69–74; 118 (June 1990): 39–44.

Bowers, Russell V. "A Confederate General Hospital: Chimborazo Post (1862–1865)." *The Scarab,* Nov. 1962, 1–5, 21.

Breeden, James O. "Confederate General Hospitals: The Front Line of the South's Civil War Health Care System." *North Carolina Medical Journal* 53, no. 2 (Feb. 1992).

Brewer, James H. *The Confederate Negro: Virginia's Craftsmen and Military Laborers, 1861–1865.* Durham, N.C.: Duke Univ. Press, 1969.

Brieger, Gert H. "Classics and Character: Medicine and Gentility." *Bulletin of the History of Medicine* 65, no. 1 (1991): 88–109.

Brock, Thomas D., Michael T. Madigan, John M. Martinko, and Jack Parker. *Biology of Microorganisms.* 7th ed. Englewood Cliffs, N.J.: Prentice Hall, 1994.

Brooks, Stewart. *Civil War Medicine.* Springfield, Ill.: Charles C. Thomas, 1966.

Bynum, W. F., and Roy Porter, eds. *Medicine and the Five Senses.* Cambridge: Cambridge Univ. Press, 1993.

Chesnut, Mary Boykin. *Mary Chesnut's Civil War.* Edited by C. Vann Woodward. New Haven, Conn.: Yale Univ. Press, 1981.

Colon, Gustavo A. "Innovative Civil War Surgeon." *Southern Medical Journal* 85, no. 4 (Apr. 1992): 411–15.

Corn, Jacqueline Karnell. "Community Responsibility For Public Health: The Impact of Epidemic Disease and Urban Growth on Pittsburgh." *Western Pennsylvania Historical Magazine* 59 (July 1976): 319–39.

Cullen, Joseph P. "Chimborazo: That Charnal House of Living Sufferers." *Civil War Times Illustrated* 29 (Jan. 1981): 36–42.

———. *Richmond Battlefields: A History and Guide to Richmond National Battlefield Park.* Washington, D.C.: National Park Service, 1992.

Cumming, Kate. *Kate: The Journal of a Confederate Nurse.* Edited by Richard Barksdale Harwell. Baton Rouge: Louisiana State Univ. Press, 1959.

Cunningham, Andrew, and Perry Williams, eds. *The Laboratory Revolution in Medicine.* Cambridge: Cambridge Univ. Press, 1992.

Cunningham, H. H. *Doctors in Gray: The Confederate Medical Service.* Baton Rouge: Louisiana State Univ. Press, 1960.

Dannett, Sylvia G. L. "Lincoln's Ladies in White." *New York State Journal of Medicine* 61 (June 1, 1961): 1944–52.

Denney, Robert E. *Civil War Medicine: Care and Comfort of the Wounded.* New York: Sterling Publishing Co., 1994.

Dowdey, Clifford. *Experiment in Rebellion.* Garden City, N.Y.: Doubleday, 1946.

Dowling, Harry F. *City Hospitals: The Undercare of the Underprivileged.* Cambridge, Mass.: Harvard Univ. Press, 1982.

———. "Politics, Medical Education and the Contagious Diseases: Sydenham Hospital of Baltimore." *Journal of the History of Medicine and Allied Sciences* 40 (Jan. 1985): 5–21.

Duffy, John. *From Humors to Medical Science: A History of American Medicine.* 2nd ed. Chicago: Univ. of Illinois Press, 1993.

———. *The Healers: The Rise of the Medical Establishment.* New York: McGraw-Hill, 1976.

———. "Medicine in the West: An Historical Overview." *Journal of the West* 21, no. 3 (July 1982): 5–14.

Duke, Maurice, and Daniel P. Jordan, eds. *A Richmond Reader: 1733–1983.* Chapel Hill: Univ. of North Carolina Press, 1983.

Ferris, Sylvia Van Voast, and Eleanor Sellers Hope. *Scalpels and Sabers: Nineteenth Century Medicine in Texas.* Austin, Tex.: Eakin, 1985.

Flint, Austin. "Conservative Medicine." In *Medical America in the Nineteenth Century: Readings from the Literature.* Edited by Gert H. Brieger. Baltimore: Johns Hopkins Univ. Press, 1972.

Franke, Norman H. "Official and Industrial Aspects of Pharmacy in the Confederacy." *Georgia Historical Quarterly* 37 (fall 1953): 175–87.

———. "Pharmaceutical Conditions and Drug Supply in the Confederacy." *Georgia Historical Quarterly* 37 (winter 1953): 287–98.

———. "Pharmacy and Pharmacists in the Confederacy." *Georgia Historical Quarterly* 38 (Mar. 1954): 11–28.

Freemon, Frank R. "Administration of the Medical Department of the Confederate States Army, 1861 to 1865." *Southern Medical Journal* 80 (May 1987): 630–37.

Furgurson, Ernest B. *Ashes of Glory: Richmond at War.* New York: Alfred A. Knopf, 1996.

Gildersleeve, John R. "History of Chimborazo Hospital, Richmond, Va., and Its Medical Officers During 1861–1865." *Virginia Medical Monthly* 88, no. 10 (Oct. 1961): 586–94.

Gillett, Mary C. *The Army Medical Department, 1818–1865.* Washington, D.C.: Center of Military History, United States Army, 1987.

Gilman, Alfred Goodman, Louis S. Goodman, Theodore W. Rall, and Ferid Murad, eds. *The Pharmacological Basis of Therapeutics.* 7th ed. New York: Macmillan, 1985.

Glaab, Charles N. *The American City: A Documentary History.* Homewood, Ill.: Dorsey Press, 1963.

Goff, Richard. *Confederate Supply.* Durham, N.C.: Duke Univ. Press, 1969.

Hansen, Bert. "America's First Medical Breakthrough." *American Historical Review* 103, no. 2 (Apr. 1998): 373–418.

Helmstadter, Carol. "Robert Bentley Todd, Saint John's House, and the Origins of the Modern Trained Nurse." *Bulletin of the History of Medicine* 67, no. 2 (1993): 282–319.

Higby, Gregory J. *In Service to American Pharmacy: The Professional Life of William Procter, Jr.* Tuscaloosa: Univ. of Alabama Press, 1992.

Hindle, Brooke, ed. *America's Wooden Age: Aspects of its Early Technology.* Tarrytown, N.Y.: Sleepy Hollow Restorations, 1975.

Howell, Joel D. *Technology in the Hospital: Transforming Patient Care in the Early Twentieth Century.* Baltimore: Johns Hopkins Univ. Press, 1995.

Huddle, Thomas S. "Looking Backward: The 1871 Reforms at Harvard Medical School Reconsidered." *Bulletin of the History of Medicine* 65, no. 3 (1991): 340–65.

Hume, Edgar Erskine. "Chimborazo Hospital, Confederate States Army, America's Largest Military Hospital." *Virginia Medical Monthly* 61 (Mar. 1934): 189–95.

"James Brown McCaw, M.D." *The British Medical Journal* 2 (Sept. 8, 1906): 601.

Johns, Frank S., and Anne Page. "Chimborazo Hospital and J. B. McCaw, Surgeon In Chief." *Virginia Magazine of History and Biography* 62 (Oct. 1954): 190–200.

Karolevitz, Robert F. *Doctors of the Old West: A Pictorial History of Medicine on the Frontier.* Seattle: Superior, 1967.

Kaufman, Martin. *Homeopathy in America: The Rise and Fall of a Medical Heresy.* Baltimore: Johns Hopkins Univ. Press, 1971.

Kett, Joseph F. *The Formation of the American Medical Profession: The Role of Institutions, 1780–1860.* New Haven, Conn.: Yale Univ. Press, 1968.

Kramer, Howard D. "The Effect of the Civil War on the Public Health Movement." *The Mississippi Valley Historical Review* 35 (Dec. 1948): 449–62.

Kuhn, Thomas S. *The Structure of Scientific Revolutions.* 2nd ed. Chicago: Univ. of Chicago Press, 1970.

Kuz, Julian E., and Bradley P. Bengtson. *Orthopaedic Injuries of the Civil War: An Atlas of Orthopaedic Injuries and Treatments During the Civil War.* Kennesaw, Ga.: Kennesaw Mountain Press, 1996.

Leake, Chauncey D. *An Historical Account of Pharmacology to the Twentieth Century.* Springfield, Ill.: Charles C. Thomas, 1975.

Maher, Sister Mary Denis. *To Bind Up the Wounds: Catholic Sister Nurses in the U.S. Civil War.* New York: Greenwood, 1989.

Maxwell, William Quentin. *Lincoln's Fifth Wheel: The Political History of the United States Sanitary Commission.* New York: Longmans, Green & Co., 1956.

McPherson, James M. *Ordeal by Fire: The Civil War and Reconstruction.* New York: Alfred A. Knopf, 1982.

Mitchell, Joseph B. *Decisive Battles of the Civil War.* Greenwich, Conn.: Fawcett Publications, 1955.

Mordecai, Samuel. *Richmond in By-Gone Days.* 1860. Reprint, Richmond, Va.: Dietz Press Inc., 1940.

Nichols, James L. *The Confederate Quartermaster in the Trans-Mississippi.* Austin: Univ. of Texas Press, 1964.

Nightingale, Florence. "Notes on Nursing." In *Selected Writings of Florence Nightingale.* Edited by Lucy Ridgely Seymer. New York: Macmillan, 1954.

Nixon, Pat Ireland. *A Century of Medicine in San Antonio: The Story of Medicine in Bexar County, Texas.* San Antonio, Tex.: self-published, 1936.

Norwood, William Frederick. *Medical Education in the United States Before the Civil War.* Philadelphia: Univ. of Pennsylvania Press, 1944.

Pember, Phoebe Yates. *A Southern Woman's Story: Life in Confederate Richmond, 1862–1865.* Edited by Bell Irvin Wiley. Marietta, Ga.: Mockingbird Books, 1992.

Reverby, Susan M. *Ordered to Care: The Dilemma of American Nursing, 1850–1945.* Cambridge: Cambridge Univ. Press, 1987.

Richardson, Robert G. *The Story of Modern Surgery.* New York: Collier, 1964.

Rosenberg, Charles E. "And Heal the Sick: The Hospital and the Patient in 19th Century America." *Journal of Social History,* Mar. 1984, 428–47.

———. *The Care of Strangers: The Rise of America's Hospital System.* Baltimore: Johns Hopkins Univ. Press, 1987.

———. *The Cholera Years: The United States in 1832, 1849, and 1866.* Chicago: Univ. of Chicago Press, 1987.

Ross, Fitzgerald. *Cities and Camps of the Confederate States.* Urbana: Univ. of Illinois Press, 1958.

Rothstein, William G. *American Physicians in the Nineteenth Century: From Sects to Science.* Baltimore: Johns Hopkins Univ. Press, 1972.

Ryan, Mary P. *Cradle of the Middle Class: The Family in Oneida County, New York, 1790–1865.* Cambridge: Cambridge Univ. Press, 1981.

Saum, Lewis O. "Death in the Popular Mind of Pre–Civil War America." *American Quarterly* 26 (Dec. 1974): 477–95.

Schroeder-Lein, Glenna R. *Confederate Hospitals on the Move: Samuel H. Stout and the Army of Tennessee.* Columbia: Univ. of South Carolina Press, 1994.

Shryock, Richard Harrison. *Medicine and Society in America: 1660–1860.* New York: New York Univ. Press, 1960.

Simkins, Francis Butler, and James Welch Patton. *Women of the Confederacy.* Richmond, Va.: Garrett & Massie, 1936.

———. "The Work of Southern Women among the Sick and Wounded of the Confederate Armies." *Journal of Southern History* 1 (Nov. 1935): 475–96.

Smith, Savage. "Map of Chimborazo General Hospital, C.S.A., as it appeared July 6, 1862." *Virginia Medical Monthly* 71 (1944): 118.

Stanard, Mary Newton. *Richmond, Its People and Its Story.* Philadelphia: J. B. Lippincott Co, 1923.

Starr, Paul. *The Social Transformation of American Medicine.* New York: Basic Books, 1982.

Stark, Richard Boies. "Surgeons and Surgical Care of the Confederate States Army." *Virginia Medical Monthly* 88, no. 10 (Oct. 1961): 604–16.

Steiner, Paul E. *Disease in the Civil War: Natural Biological Warfare in 1861–65.* Springfield, Ill.: Charles C. Thomas, 1968.

Stevenson, Isobel. "American Medicine During the Sixties." *Ciba Symposia* 3 (July 1941): 894–907.

Stinson, Byron. "The Army Disease." *American History Illustrated,* Dec. 1971, 10–17.

Straubing, Harold Elk, ed. *In Hospital and Camp: The Civil War through the Eyes of Its Doctors and Nurses.* Harrisburg, Pa.: Stackpole Books, 1993.

Tebault, Christopher H. "Hospitals of the Confederacy." *Southern Practitioner* 24 (1902): 499–509.

Thompson, W. T., Jr., and E. Randolph Trice. "The Man of the Hour." *The Scarab,* Nov. 1962, 6, 21.

Townsend, Gavin. "Airborne Toxins and the American House, 1865–1895." *Winterthur Portfolio: A Journal of American Material Culture* 24 (Spring 1989): 29–42.

Vogel, Morris J. *The Invention of the Modern Hospital: Boston, 1870–1930.* Chicago: Univ. of Chicago Press, 1980.

Waitt, Robert W. *Confederate Military Hospitals in Richmond.* Official Publication No. 22, Richmond Civil War Centennial Committee. Richmond, Va.: City of Richmond, 1964.

Ward, Patricia Spain. *Simon Baruch: Rebel in the Ranks of Medicine, 1840–1921.* Tuscaloosa: Univ. of Alabama Press, 1994.

Warner, John Harley. "A Southern Medical Reform: The Meaning of the Antebellum Argument for Southern Education." *Bulletin of the History of Medicine* 57, no. 3 (1983): 364–81.

————. *The Therapeutic Perspective: Medical Practice, Knowledge, and Identity in America, 1820–1885.* Cambridge, Mass.: Harvard Univ. Press, 1986.

Warthen, Harry J. "Confederate Medicine, 1861–1865." *Virginia Medical Monthly* 88, no. 10 (Oct. 1961): 573–75.

Welsh, Jack D. *Medical Histories of Confederate Generals.* Kent, Ohio: Kent State Univ. Press, 1995.

Welch, Spencer Glasgow. *A Confederate Surgeon's Letters to His Wife.* Marietta, Ga.: Continental, 1954.

Williams, Carrington. "Samuel Preston Moore: Surgeon General of the Confederate States Army." *Virginia Medical Monthly* 88, no. 10 (Oct. 1961): 622–28.

Wood, Ann Douglas. "The War Within a War: Women Nurses in the Union Army." *Civil War History* 18 (Sept. 1972): 197–212.

Wylie, W. Gill. *Hospitals: Their History, Organization and Construction.* New York: Appleton, 1877.

UNPUBLISHED DISSERTATIONS, THESES, AND CONFERENCE PAPERS

Ballou, Charles F. "Hospital Medicine in Richmond, Virginia during the Civil War: A Study of Hospital No. 21, Howard's Grove, and Winder Hospitals." Master's thesis, Virginia Polytechnic Institute and State Univ., 1992.

Bollet, Alfred J. "How Good or Bad Was Medical Care during the Civil War?" Presentation at the National Museum of Civil War Medicine, Fredericksburg, Md., Aug. 1995.

Bruegmann, Robert. "Architecture of the Hospital: 1770–1870, Design and Technology." Ph.D. diss., Univ. of Pennsylvania, 1976.

Cook, Charles. "Chimborazo Hospital: Flagship Medical Center of the Confederacy." Presentation at the National Museum of Civil War Medicine Conference, Aug. 1995.

Irby, Gloria R. "Chimborazo and Lincoln Hospitals." Master's thesis, Humboldt State College, 1967.

Smith, Nina Bennett. "The Women Who Went to the War: The Union Army Nurse in the Civil War." Ph.D. diss., Northwestern Univ., 1981.

Sokolowsky, William. "The Military Hospitals in the Washington, D.C. Area During the Civil War." Master's thesis, George Washington Univ., 1958.

INDEX

Chimborazo was designed and typeset on a Macintosh computer system using QuarkXPress software. The body text and display type are set in 9/13 Stone Serif. This book was designed and typeset by Barbara Karwhite and manufactured by Thomson-Shore, Inc.